A Therapist's Guide to Neurodiversity Affirming Practice with Children and Young People

A Therapist's Guide to
Neurodiversity Affirming Practice
with Children and Young People

Raelene Dundon

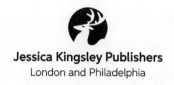

Jessica Kingsley Publishers
London and Philadelphia

First published in Great Britain in 2024 by Jessica Kingsley Publishers
An imprint of John Murray Press

2

Copyright © Raelene Dundon 2024

The right of Raelene Dundon to be identified as the Author of the Work has been
asserted by her in accordance with the Copyright, Designs and Patents Act 1988.

Front cover image source: Shutterstock®.

Content Warning: This book mentions anxiety, suicidal ideation, and trauma.

A CIP catalogue record for this title is available from the
British Library and the Library of Congress.

ISBN 978 1 83997 585 1
eISBN 978 1 83997 586 8

Printed and bound by CPI Group (UK) Ltd, Croydon, CR0 4YY

Jessica Kingsley Publishers' policy is to use papers that are natural, renewable
and recyclable products and made from wood grown in sustainable
forests. The logging and manufacturing processes are expected to conform
to the environmental regulations of the country of origin.

Jessica Kingsley Publishers
Carmelite House
50 Victoria Embankment
London EC4Y 0DZ

www.jkp.com

John Murray Press
Part of Hodder & Stoughton Limited
An Hachette UK Company

For my Neurokin

Contents

Acknowledgments

This book is something I have wanted to write for a while, and making it a reality has only been possible through the support and guidance of some very special people.

First, as always, to my wonderful husband Andrew. Thank you for always being there as a sounding board, a proofreader, a cheerleader, and a voice of reason. I could not have done this without you.

To Jo, Carla, and Jodie, all clinicians I highly respect and whose friendship I value. Thank you for giving your time and knowledge to review my drafts and for helping me make this book the very best that it could be.

A special thank you to my friend Yael Clark, neurodivergent psychologist, for her insights and knowledge of neurodiversity affirming practice, and for helping me navigate my way as a neurodivergent clinician. Your encouragement and guidance has been invaluable.

Thank you to Chloe for sharing her perspective and expertise as a multiply neurodivergent teen, and for trusting me to share her voice to help advocate for others. And thank you to Kiah for her insights and for allowing me to be part of her journey.

Finally, thank you to the neurodivergent community, and in particular my neurodivergent clients, colleagues, friends, and family. I am grateful to have you in my life, and will continue to value the opportunity to learn and grow with you as we continue to advocate for a better future for all of us.

A Note to Readers

Throughout this book, you will notice that I have primarily used identity-first language (e.g., Autistic, Dyslexic, ADHDer, neurodivergent) when referring to children and adolescents rather than using person-first language (e.g., person with Autism). I have done this because a large part of the neurodivergent community prefer identity-first language as they see their neurodivergence as integral to who they are as individuals, and they feel that person-first language implies a defect or disorder that they do not relate to.

Although I understand that there will be some members of the neurodivergent community who prefer person-first language, and individual preferences should always be respected, using identity-first language is generally considered more consistent with a neurodiversity affirming approach, and so this book is written in a style that best reflects that.

I am also aware that many of you, as clinicians, will have been trained to use person-first language in your work, so seeing identity-first language being used in a book may feel uncomfortable and seem "wrong." I am hopeful that by the end of this book you will feel more comfortable with identity-first language, and be confident to use it with your clients and the wider community.

I would also like to mention that this book has been written for medical professionals, allied health professionals, and any other clinicians working with children and adolescents. So, to capture the diverse nature of the professional community this book is intended to inform, I have used the terms "therapist" and "clinician" inter-changeably throughout.

Introduction

Thank you to everyone for taking the time to read this book.

I want to start by giving you an idea of what being a neurodiversity affirming parent and clinician means to me. There are different definitions about what neurodiversity affirming is, but for me, the heart of it is understanding that there is natural variation in brain types across the human population, and all types of brains are important and valuable. This means that neurodivergent brains (brains that vary from what is considered "normal") should be seen as natural and equally as important, rather than as disordered. When we do this, we can unconditionally accept neurodivergent individuals for who they are, and celebrate and accommodate their differences by providing individualized supports that meet their specific needs.

I think it's important to recognize that while there will be many people reading this book who feel empowered by new knowledge, and others who will feel like their understanding and approach to neurodivergence has been validated, many of us may also feel a sense of shame or guilt or regret for how we have parented our children, taught our students, supported our clients, or even for what we have expected from ourselves before we had this knowledge. I can't tell you not to feel this way, but I want you to remember that we all make mistakes, we are all doing the best we can with the information we have, and if we discover that what we have been doing is not helpful, or has even been harmful, we can now make a change.

When I was studying psychology over 20 years ago, the way we understood and learned about neurotypes such as Autism and ADHD (Attention-Deficit Hyperactivity Disorder) was through the medical model. Recommended supports were behavioral in nature, focusing on changing a child's behavior to make them conform to typical standards and comply with adult direction and instruction. Unfortunately, all this time later, psychology students continue to be taught within this behavioral framework, and it is the same across training for educators, allied health professionals, and parents and caregivers.[1] But change is happening, and you are part of that change.

As a parent of Autistic children who are now young adults, I can look back and see lots of mistakes. It is a confronting thing to acknowledge that you have done something that may have caused distress to a loved one, especially when you had the best of intentions, but with acknowledgment comes the possibility of change and the opportunity for healing. I have been able to say sorry to my children for some of my mistakes. Like not allowing one of my boys to wear earplugs in noisy situations because I wanted him to "get used to it." I wasn't aware at the time that sensory sensitivities shouldn't be addressed in this way, and so when he wanted to put his earplugs in, I would tell him to wait a bit, so he was exposed to the sound before putting them in. This caused him distress because I wasn't understanding how serious this was for him, and I was subjecting him to sensory input that hurt his ears. The revelation that this had been the wrong thing to do weighed heavily on me, but I was able to talk to my son about it and apologize for not understanding his needs and the hurt I'd caused. We may not all be able to have discussions like this with our loved ones or our clients, but we can show others that we recognize the need to do better by being open to new ideas and changing our approach to be more accepting and affirming. In time, we can hopefully move forward and leave those mistakes behind.

When I was starting my family in the early 2000s, I was also

---

1   Where I refer to parents throughout the book, I also mean caregivers.

finishing my studies and beginning my career in psychology, so as I have grown as a parent over the years, I have also grown as a clinician.

I count myself lucky that at the start of my career I worked in early childhood services with children who presented with a range of developmental differences. Because of the nature of my work, the supports offered were very family-centered and play-based. While there are certainly methods that were used then that I would not use now, my work did not involve more strict behavioral intervention. I did, however, use the typical behavior management tools of the time, which included reward charts and implementing consequences to facilitate behavior changes. I didn't know any different.

As I gained experience and worked with more children and families, there were times when I questioned what I had learned and how applicable it was to my practice. However, there wasn't always a clear path to new or different information, and research was limited.

The thing about being open to ongoing learning is that when you find an answer to a question about something, one thing can lead to another, and you often end up with even more unanswered questions.

What I started to discover was that assumptions were being made that children who were behaving in similar ways must be doing so for the same reasons, and this didn't make sense to me. I could see that each child's individual sensitivities, needs, and experiences impacted on how they would interact with their environment and why they might respond in particular ways to different situations. So, for example, just because two children were distressed when sitting at the table for snack time didn't mean that the reason for their distress would be the same. This was when my journey to neurodiversity affirming practice really started, but I didn't know it back then.

Over the last decade or so, I have learned from professionals such as Dr. Ross Greene, Dr. Dan Siegel, Dr. Bruce Perry, Alfie Kohn, Dr. Stuart Shanker and Bo Hejlskov Elvén, as well as lived experience experts, and what I have learned has changed my work and my life.

I have increased my understanding of the stress response and how regulation, connection, and safety impacts a child's ability to learn, how the development of self-regulation relies on co-regulation, the importance of interoception, why presuming competence is essential, and how child-led and non-directive approaches can support autonomy. But I still have a lot to learn.

There have been many moments over the years that have shaped my practice and parenting in positive ways, and many of them have occurred when something didn't feel right, and I questioned it. I have had many conversations with parents, educators, and clinicians who have experienced the same thing—many who doubt themselves because someone in authority has told them to do something and they think they shouldn't question it. But today I would encourage you to do just that. For example, if you see a clinician ask a parent to trigger a child's meltdown so they can observe it, or to create a situation that causes the child distress so they can practice calming down, ask them why. If something about what you are being asked to do doesn't feel right, ask for more information or research or another opinion. You have the power to take a different path.

I would like to take a moment here to especially encourage clinicians to think about the type of therapist they want to be, and to be open to changing the way they support their neurodivergent clients. It is easy to get stuck in a certain way of practicing that we are familiar with, and we think is effective, but the reality is that one size does not fit all. We need to be flexible and tailor our supports to every client's individual needs. Just because a particular approach is "evidence-based" or the way it's always been done doesn't mean it's right. Questioning and having a deeper understanding of why we do what we do will make us better therapists and allow us to provide more affirming and effective supports to our neurodivergent clients.

I feel lucky that I have been able to take a different path and embrace a new way of seeing neurodivergence and supporting neurodivergent children and families, but it is still a work in progress. Making changes to my practice and my parenting has been ongoing, and I am learning constantly. Being an author and a presenter has also meant that my journey has been quite public. While I have always been an advocate for the neurodivergent community, I didn't always get it right. For example, five years ago I was still presenting seminars on "work refusal and noncompliance" that included rewards and consequences, and three years ago I wrote a social skills curriculum for Autistic children—which, on reflection, was focused mostly on teaching neurotypical social skills. The important thing for me is that I am continuing to learn and grow and share my new knowledge, even if it means admitting that I have been wrong in the past.

I am also still early in my own journey of discovery as a late-diagnosed Autistic ADHDer, and with that comes reflection and a reexamination of my past experiences through a lens of difference rather than one of feeling flawed and less than my peers, particularly when I couldn't meet neurotypical standards in my work and personal life. Even with this realization, I find myself regularly battling the internalized ableism of expecting that I should be able to do things that others can do without support, and at times feeling ashamed that I need to get help. I truly believe that embracing the idea of neurodiversity and supporting children in neurodiversity affirming ways will help the next generation of neurodivergent children to flourish without them having to question their self-worth or abilities.

I do understand how hard it can be to approach supporting children in a different way. Colleagues may tell you that what you are doing is not "evidence-based" or that a child needs to learn what the "real world" is like. But they don't have the knowledge that you do. I hope that what you learn in the following pages will give you the courage to start to make positive change in whatever way you are able.

For those of you who are further along in your journey to being neurodiversity affirming, please remember that you were once new to this concept, just like the many who are hearing about this idea for the first time. It is important that whenever we can, we welcome questions, acknowledge the courage it takes to make change, and be understanding of the inevitable mistakes people will make along the way. And for those new to the ideas that have been presented here, please remember that many of us have experienced trauma and have lived a lifetime of being misunderstood and mistreated due to our neurodivergence, so how you respond to us sharing our experiences and advice is important.

One of the most dangerous phrases in history would have to be "but we've always done it that way." With what we know now about neurodiversity and how best to support neurodivergent individuals, now is the time to make sure we don't go back to practices that we know cause trauma and distress.

So thank you for reading this book and being open to change. I hope it supports you in your journey towards neurodiversity affirming practice. Even a small change can make a big difference.

— PART 1 —

IN THEORY

— Chapter 1 —

What Is Neurodiversity?

The term "neurodiversity" was first introduced in the 1990s by Judith Singer to describe the natural variation in human brain development resulting in differences in cognition, communication, perception, and behavior (see Singer 2017).

While the idea of human brains being naturally varied in their development may not seem like a big deal, the concept really revolutionized the way many saw neurodevelopmental conditions, and was the beginning of the neurodiversity affirming movement that has largely become a human rights initiative.

Historically, disorders have been defined by how the characteristic behaviors associated with that condition differ from what is considered "normal," and how an individual is impaired by those characteristics. In essence, the presence of a disorder indicates that someone is a faulty or broken version of a "normal" person.

The reason that the idea of neurodiversity is so important is that it suggests that rather than being broken, individuals whose brain development and function differs from the norm are just different. The neurodiversity affirming movement takes that one step further to suggest that we should accept and support all these brain differences rather than stigmatize or pathologize them.

From within the concept of neurodiversity come the terms "neurotypical" or "neuronormative" and "neurodivergent." As the terms suggest, "neuronormative" or "neurotypical" brains are the majority—they are brain types that are considered "normal" due to the frequency of their occurrence in the general population. In contrast, "neurodivergent," a term coined by Kassiane Asasumasu (neurodivergent writer and advocate), refers to individuals whose brains diverge or differ from the norm in terms of their neurology (see Chapman 2021).

When Asasumasu first introduced the term "neurodivergent," she stated that it should be considered a tool of inclusion in which anyone with different neurology from the majority should be included. She suggested that neurotypes such as Autism, ADHD, Obsessive-Compulsive Disorder (OCD), Intellectual Disability, Post-Traumatic Stress Disorder (PTSD), Developmental Trauma, and Learning Disabilities, as well as medical conditions such as epilepsy, cerebral palsy, and Parkinson's disease, and mental health conditions such as anxiety and depression, should all be considered neurodivergent as they all involve differences in brain structure or function.

However, there continues to be much discussion regarding the neurotypes that should be included within the term "neurodivergent" and those that should not, perhaps due to it being possible to be born neurodivergent or to acquire neurodivergence due to trauma, injury, or disease. It is also possible to be "multiply neurodivergent," a term used to describe individuals whose neurotype differs from the norm in more than one way.

One description I have read that attempts to distinguish between these different types of neurodivergences is by Dr. Nick Walker, a queer, transgender, Autistic writer and educator who is known for her work in the neurodiversity space. Dr. Walker describes innate neurodivergences such as Autism, ADHD, and Dyslexia as being part of an individual's self and how they relate to the world. As such they cannot and should not be separated from the person or "treated" in an effort to eradicate them. In contrast, she describes other forms of neurodivergence, such as epilepsy or Parkinson's disease, as being separate to an individual's self, as the removal of the medical symptoms would not result in a fundamental change in who the individual is. Further, in some cases an individual may seek out treatment or support to cure them, particularly when there are medical implications.

Perhaps another way of considering this is to think about individuals who see their neurodivergence as part of their identity, and as such would not want to have it taken away, and others who see their neurodivergence as something that has a negative impact on their life, and would be happy to have it taken away if they could. And then there may be those multiply neurodivergent individuals who accept parts of who they are as their identity, but would like to see other parts removed to improve their quality of life. This is not a black and white issue, and an individual's feelings about their neurodivergence may change from day to day. Regardless, I believe an individual's attitude towards their own neurodivergence, whatever it may be and however they identify with it, needs to be respected.

In future chapters, I will be focusing primarily on how we can support neurodivergent children and adolescents within the neurodiversity affirming framework, as neurotypical children generally already receive affirming supports when seeking therapy but neurodivergent children historically may not. Also, when discussing neurodivergence, I will be referring mainly to neurotypes generally considered innate and part of an individual's identity, such as Autism, ADHD, Learning Disabilities, Tourette's syndrome, and Down syndrome. These neurodivergent individuals may require support and accommodations to manage some of their challenges (e.g., with respect to neurotypical societal rules and expectations or health conditions), but would generally not want to change who they are.

I am aware that this definition of neurodivergence will not resonate with everyone, and I am conscious of being respectful and considerate towards all viewpoints. However, the broader issues around identity and neurodivergence are too big for me to attempt to resolve here. Ultimately, the way an individual sees their neurodivergence depends on their own personal journey and experiences. But all neurodivergent individuals deserve to be treated with respect and dignity, and to be supported to access the same opportunities as the neurotypical population, and that is what being neurodiversity affirming is about.

— Chapter 2 —

What Does It Mean to Be Neurodiversity Affirming?

Being neurodiversity affirming is not just about following a set of rules or recommendations that you use some of the time; it is about a philosophy that guides the whole of your practice with every client.

At its heart is the basic human right that all people deserve to be treated with respect and have their needs met. This may seem blatantly obvious, and it certainly should be something that doesn't need to be mentioned, but time and time again I have seen members of the disabled community in general treated as "less than" by the professionals who are supposed to support and advocate for them. I believe that most clinicians have the best of intentions, but when they make assumptions about the client's wants and needs and don't provide them with the opportunity to have whatever input they can into their own therapy and supports, they are taking away their client's autonomy and not offering them the respect that another person would normally expect to receive.

To be neurodiversity affirming is to acknowledge that all neuro-types, even those who differ from the norm, are equal in value and valid in their right to exist. This means that we value an individual's strengths and accommodate their challenges. It also means that we accept differences in communication, social interaction, behavior, and learning.

One way that we can start to shift our thinking about disability and neurodiversity to a more affirming philosophy is to move away from the more traditional medical model of disability towards a social model.

The medical model of disability focuses on symptoms and cures and defines conditions in terms of deficits and disorders. This is the traditional way that disability, and indeed neurodivergence, has been viewed, and extends from the idea of an impaired or broken "normal" person. If someone is functioning in a different way to the norm, they are viewed as needing to be fixed.

This may be the case for medical conditions that are life limiting and that impact health and quality of life, such as diseases and serious mental health conditions. However, many feel that this should not be extended to neurodivergence such as being Autistic, ADHD, and Dyslexic, with the premise that just because someone differs from the norm doesn't mean there is something wrong with them.

The problem is that society has a history of pathologizing any behavior or presentation that is different to the norm or not understood. In doing so, they alienate and stigmatize individuals whose differences make it challenging for them to function within society's default expectations, instead of recognizing that in many cases it's the role of society to support the needs of the individual. This is where the social model of disability comes in.

The social model of disability focuses on individuals being disabled by their environment, and a lack of understanding and accommodations impacting on their ability to function. It recognizes differences in skills such as social interaction, communication, thinking, and behavior rather than deficits, and in this way is consistent with the idea of being neurodiversity affirming.

Within this model, environmental adaptations can reduce or remove the level of disability an individual experiences. For example, an individual in a wheelchair would have significant difficulty entering a building that was only accessible via stairs when other people who were ambulant would not have that difficulty. However, if there was a ramp at the building, people in wheelchairs and ambulant individuals would all have equal access. Therefore, with a ramp in place, the wheelchair user would be just as able as others to enter the building.

This idea can be further extended to not just consider adaptations to the physical environment, but also to the social environment.

A TEDx talk in 2019 by Jac den Houting, an Autistic researcher in Australia, explains this concept in relation to the Autistic neurotype brilliantly. They encourage the community to view being Autistic as a cultural difference, one in which different ways of communicating and behaving should be accepted and supported by the neurotypical population. For example, when interacting with someone from another country, where there may be language and cultural differences, we would usually make allowances for differences in the way they communicate and interact, and adapt our own communication style to support them to understand and feel comfortable. However, this tends not to occur when neurotypical individuals interact with Autistic individuals. Instead, the Autistic individual's communication and social interaction skills are labeled as impaired, and there is often an expectation on the Autistic person to learn how to communicate like their neurotypical peers.

This idea is further highlighted by the "double empathy problem" introduced by Autistic researcher Dr. Damian Milton. He proposes that the social and communication difficulties that are considered a feature of Autism are caused by a disconnect between Autistic and neurotypical communication styles due to a lack of mutual understanding and reciprocity, not a social deficit in Autistic individuals. This then suggests that the responsibility of communicating successfully is on both parties, not just the Autistic individual.

Similar arguments could be made for many other neurodivergent neurotypes. For example, if children were given flexible sitting options in the classroom, would an ADHDer be disabled by their need to move? Or if children were able to demonstrate their knowledge and learning in a variety of creative ways other than just producing an essay, would a Dysgraphic child be disabled by their difficulty with writing?

When we approach neurodivergence and disability through an affirming lens, we can see an individual's strengths and challenges, and explore how to support them to remove social and environmental barriers and live the life they want to live, with the same opportunities as their neurotypical peers.

A NOTE ABOUT NEURODIVERGENCE AND DISABILITY

I feel that it is important to note that for many neurodivergent individuals, embracing their differences does not mean that they do not consider themselves disabled in some way. It means that they accept themselves as they are and recognize their strengths, as well as acknowledging that they have challenges that require supports. They also understand that with the appropriate supports and accommodations in place, they will be less impacted by their challenges and more able to do the things they want to do.

I should also mention here that the notion of disability and being disabled is very individual, and while many neurodivergent individuals identify as being disabled, there are also members of the neurodivergent community who do not identify this way at all. As with most concepts discussed within this book, it is important to respect individual ideas, perspectives, and preferences, and to work with clients in whatever way they are most comfortable with, and in a way that they can relate to.

Chapter 3

Why Are Changes in Therapeutic Practice Needed?

Since starting my career as a psychologist 20 years ago, there are many aspects of the profession that have changed, but also many that have concerningly stayed the same. I have found this to be true of most of the helping professions, whether that is in medicine or allied health. In many cases, it seems to be driven by a lack of flexibility and acceptance of change, both in the training of professionals and in clinical practice.

Now I am not saying that doctors should just start prescribing medication off label due to the latest fad, or that therapists should start using a technique they heard about online because a couple of people said it worked for them or a celebrity endorsed it. But we do have a responsibility as therapists to be open to considering and evaluating new theories and techniques, rather than being stuck teaching and using outdated information from decades ago because someone said it was the "gold standard" or "because that is the way it has always been done."

Research into the brain and body has exploded in recent years, and with it has come a greater understanding of many important aspects of our work including behavior, communication, sensory processing, emotions, and cognition. There has also been a rise in awareness and recognition of human rights, especially in marginalized populations such as the disabled community.

Unfortunately, many misconceptions continue to persist, resulting in disabled individuals, including neurodivergent individuals, having unfair and inaccurate judgments placed on them that impact the way they are treated by health professionals and the wider community.

For example, the tendency for health professionals to speak to carers and not directly to individuals with a disability, treating them like they are invisible, appears to continue to be far more common than it should be in this day and age. There still seems to be an assumption in many health professions, and certainly in the wider community, that having a visible disability equates to a person being unable to think or understand what is happening around them, which is offensive in the least and discriminatory at worst. Then there is the common assumption that an individual who is Autistic and/or has an Intellectual Disability and is minimally speaking can't understand what is being said about them or contribute to their own care. These assumptions can be damaging and can violate the client's rights.

Further, there continues to be a persistent opinion in the disability sector that individuals with a disability somehow don't deserve to be treated with the same dignity and respect that would be offered to other people.

For example, I have seen recommendations from internationally recognized services that suggest individuals who have experienced trauma should receive person-centered and trauma-informed supports, but Autistic individuals need behavioral interventions. I have spoken to numerous clients and their families who have been told by therapists that they are not working hard enough or doing enough to see improvement, when the therapists themselves just use the same methods with every client they see, regardless of that client's presentation and needs, and expect to see change. And I have consoled more children than I can count who have been punished for their differences, and told that they just need to try harder or make better choices about things that are physiologically and cognitively beyond their control.

As clinicians, we need to do better.

One change that is essential is to separate the intention of therapy from how it is applied. While it is reasonable to assume that most therapeutic approaches have been designed with the intention of helping people, and certainly clinicians entering the allied health and medical professions usually do so because they want to make the lives of their clients better, having good intentions does not justify doing harm, even when it is inadvertent.

Now this is certainly not about shaming clinicians who have used approaches in the past that they were taught were effective and "best practice" and that have since been identified as potentially harmful. It is about recognizing that we have access to more research, more scientific understanding, and more reports from real people who have experienced these therapies, and we need to use this information to become better clinicians. Personally, I consider myself a lifelong learner, and I believe that being open to learning at any stage in my career is essential for me to continue to support my clients. I have always said that if there ever comes a time when I think I know everything, it will be time for me to stop practicing, because if I think I know everything, then I will not be an effective clinician.

Let's take corporal punishment in schools as an example. It really was not that long ago that the accepted way to manage and deter "inappropriate behavior" and "disrespect" in the classroom was to hit children with a stick or strap. Thankfully, the suggestion that this form of discipline be used now would be met with fierce opposition from most people. It violates the rights of the child, and has been shown to be physically and psychologically harmful. But it took many years of questioning, listening, research, and advocacy to have changes officially made in education settings, and to shift the thinking of teachers who were originally taught that using such harsh discipline was the best way to teach children how to respect adults, follow instructions, and learn, to prepare them for adulthood. For most educators of that time, the intention behind corporal punishment was arguably good—they were setting their students up for future success. However, understanding why it was done and the intention behind it doesn't make it right to continue its use. We know better now, and so we can do better.

Of equal importance in this discussion is the issue of effectiveness versus harm.

Effectiveness as an outcome usually has an association with something positive. It means that a particular treatment or method had the intended result. But what if the treatment and outcome are not in the best interests of the client? What if the therapy is effective in achieving the desired result, but in turn it causes the client harm? Should we continue with a therapy approach if we know it is harmful just because it works?

Taking the example of corporal punishment again, many parents in past generations may have said that smacking was an effective behavior management tool for their children. Some would still say that it is effective, especially if they were parented that way themselves. And if they are talking about the outcome of a child doing what they are told and not "misbehaving," then yes, it may be that smacking has been effective. However, we need to ask, at what cost? Apart from the physical harm that smacking causes, there is the constant fear in anticipation of being smacked, and the ruptured and inconsistent relationship with a parent who says they love the child but then hurts them, as well as the potential trauma carried on into adulthood. Is having a compliant child really worth that?

So, when we are considering therapeutic approaches with children, even when a therapy has been shown to be effective, we need to ask ourselves, "What is the cost to this client?"

If the cost is time and effort and the benefits are new skills and a better quality of life, it is likely that the approach is worth considering. If, however, the cost is emotional distress, fear and anxiety, or low self-esteem and self-worth, then we are doing something wrong. This is not what therapy should be about.

Consider this example: a child is being taught to complete a puzzle by repeatedly practicing the placement of puzzle pieces. When they get distressed, they are made to continue with the activity. If they try to get up and move away, they are physically forced to sit down, which causes them more distress. Eventually they finish the puzzle and are given a reward.

This may be considered "effective" therapy as the child achieved the required outcome of finishing the puzzle; however, the cost was having their distress and needs ignored, which could have lasting psychological impacts. Just because an approach has been deemed to be effective by research or clinicians doesn't mean it should be used.

EVIDENCE-BASED PRACTICE

But what about "evidence-based therapies," you may ask. If a therapy has been shown to be effective in research, doesn't that mean it will be safe to use? And shouldn't we only use therapies that are evidence-based in our practice?

Certainly, the idea of engaging in evidence-based practice is one that most clinicians are taught to strive for. Working in ways that have been researched and shown to be effective in obtaining positive outcomes for clients is at the heart of what we do. Understandably, then, when being introduced to neurodiversity affirming approaches to therapy and being told that some established approaches may be harmful to the neurodivergent community, clinicians may be concerned about whether affirming approaches are considered evidence-based. They may be reluctant to engage in new or alternative methods or supporting clients without "proof" that they are effective.

The problem with the idea of "evidence-based practice" is that not all evidence is created equal. True, evidence-based practice not only considers clinical research but also other factors regarding the suitability of an approach to an individual and the context in which the therapy is taking place.

When learning about evidence-based practice in university courses and clinician training, three parts are usually presented:

- research (evidence)
- clinical experience or expert opinion
- client and carer perspectives and needs.

All parts are important in determining the best course of action in supporting a client.

However, clinicians often get stuck on the research (evidence) part and forget that one size does not fit all in therapy. Just because an approach has clinical research to support it doesn't mean it is going to be the best thing for your clients. Similarly, just because an emerging approach has limited clinical research to support it doesn't mean it is the wrong approach or that it is not evidence-based.

I think it is important to consider all these parts in detail to discuss the strengths and limitations of evidence-based practice when working with the neurodivergent community.

RESEARCH (EVIDENCE)

When we think of research for clinical practice, we usually think about therapeutic methods that have been investigated and found to be effective in treating a particular condition. But how often do we question the way the research was conducted, who the subjects were, and what the outcomes mean?

While as clinicians it is important to keep up with current research to stay informed about new developments in our field and to critically evaluate approaches, in reality, I have found that research is often years behind clinical practice, and often tells us what we already know or at least suspect from a clinical perspective. This doesn't mean, of course, that research is not important—it definitely is. However, we need to be critical in how we interpret findings from such research, and how we adapt those findings into clinical practice.

One of the difficulties with current research is the lack of studies focused on neurodivergent individuals and their needs. Historically, research on neurodivergence, such as the Autistic neurotype, has been focused on "curing" or "reducing symptoms." Approaches were seen as effective if they resulted in an individual seeming to be "less Autistic." Because of this focus, studies into supports for Autistic individuals to combat the distress caused by mental health conditions such as anxiety, or to provide useful accommodations to individuals with ADHD in the classroom, were few and far between. Thankfully some of this research is now being done in collaboration with the neurodivergent community, but we have a long way to go.

Another problem with relying solely on research to inform therapy is that until recently, very few therapeutic approaches have been specifically designed for the neurodivergent population. Instead, approaches created and found to be effective in supporting neurotypical individuals are often used with the neurodivergent community without consideration of the fundamental differences evident between the neurotypes. This does not mean that these approaches can never be used with neurodivergent individuals, but we need to adapt them to cater to the differences in thinking, processing, perception, and learning that are evident in different neurotypes, and research into this is still in its early stages.

Finally, as I mentioned earlier, not all research is created equal, and as such the claim of being "evidence-based" can be extremely misleading. I have seen "evidence-based" programs advertised that are supported only by the creator's own research studies that would not stand up to any serious investigation. And others that have been rigorously researched and shown to be effective, although the outcomes are not affirming or beneficial to the individuals the program is supposed to support.

When we incorporate research into our practice, it is important that we are scientific and critical in our consideration of research methods. We need to be curious about not just what the research tells us, but also what it does not.

CLINICAL EXPERIENCE OR EXPERT OPINION

Clinical experience and expertise are often overlooked in the discussion of evidence-based practice, but these actually form an essential part of the concept. We need to not only understand the research, but also have an idea of how it transfers to working with real people if we are going to be effective practitioners.

As clinicians, we are expected to have a certain minimum level of expertise in our area of practice based on our training and qualifications; however, neurodivergence still attracts little focus in most clinical training. When supporting neurodivergent individuals, we often need to learn through experience and seek out additional learning to provide the best support possible. But where do we find the best information to support our clinical practice?

In recent years, the voices of neurodivergent individuals have become more prominent by sharing their lived experience of being neurodivergent to broaden the knowledge of clinicians and the general community alike. Autistics were probably the most vocal at first, and now ADHDers, Dyslexics, and others are also being heard and are sharing their strengths and challenges and their hopes for acceptance and understanding.

While the experience of one person on its own may not mirror the experience of all, each individual experience recounted is valid and important in its own right. And when those individual stories share important elements, we need to take even more notice. It is no longer enough to base our knowledge on reports from others about the neurodivergent community or engage in practice informed by research alone. It is now time to listen to the real experts, those who know neurodivergence best because they live it. We become better clinicians for being open to listening and learning, and this knowledge can then form part of true evidence-based practice.

Of course, there are many clinicians out there who claim to be experts in neurodivergence, and while some will have extensive knowledge and experience in supporting the neurodivergent community, many others know only what they have learned from books.

Clinicians with true expertise in neurodivergence have usually spent many years working with neurodivergent clients. They have grown and adapted their practice over the years in keeping with new information and understanding, and they recognize the importance of neurodivergent voices and incorporate this knowledge into their work.

There are also an increasing number of neurodivergent clinicians across medical and allied health fields who are open about their neurodivergence, and who are actively using the combination of their own lived experience and professional expertise to increase understanding and promote affirming practice among their colleagues. However, this is not something that all neurodivergent clinicians feel safe to do due to the stigma that still surrounds Autism and ADHD in particular.

Seeking to learn from those with lived experience and allies of the neurodivergent community (those who are informed by neurodivergent voices and act in keeping with the wants and needs of the neurodivergent population) is essential to effectively support your neurodivergent clients.

CLIENT AND CARER PERSPECTIVES AND NEEDS

The third piece of evidence-based practice is the consideration of client and carer perspectives and needs.

It is important that when we are supporting clients on an individual level, our approach is tailored to individual need. One size does not fit all.

Too often in my work I see clinicians applying the same approaches to individuals who may present with the same neurotype but who are vastly different in their needs, and it is expected that these approaches will be effective. There are so many factors that influence what treatment, support, or accommodation is appropriate for a client. Demographic factors such as age, gender, religion, ethnicity, and socioeconomic status may inform the appropriateness of a particular approach. Medical conditions and current medications and treatments also contribute. When the client is a child, the family and other supports around the child need to be considered, such as if there are other siblings with a disability or medical needs, parental disability and mental health, and the child's education setting. Then there are the wishes of the client and their family that should be carefully considered.

I find that in the medical profession, more consideration is often given to finding a treatment or support that individually works for a client rather than giving everyone the same medication and expecting it to work; however, in the allied health space this is not always the case, and it really needs to change.

When we consider theoretical frameworks and research findings, lived experience, and clinical expertise, as well as a client's individual wants and needs when formulating a plan to support a client, we are using true evidence-based practice to inform our approach, and as such we are much more likely to effectively meet our client's needs.

— Chapter 4 —

What Are the Principles of Neurodiversity Affirming Practice?

As we have already discussed, being neurodiversity affirming means being accepting of all neurotypes and adapting our practice to make it more accessible and effective for everyone. We can start to do this by being guided by some key principles that have been identified as being important in working in a neurodiversity affirming way.

1. PRESUME COMPETENCE

When working with clients from a neurodiversity affirming approach, it is essential that we presume competence. Presuming competence essentially means assuming that an individual can learn, think, and understand, even when we may not have concrete evidence to confirm this. When we presume competence, we are acknowledging an individual's potential, providing them with opportunities to grow and develop with whatever support they may need, and we are not limiting their experiences based on judgments about what their capabilities are.

Presuming competence sets us up to have high expectations for the children and adolescents we work with, and ensures that we offer them the same respect that we would give to any individual in our care. It also gives clients the opportunity to show us what they are capable of with the right supports in place, and we can adjust our expectations and supports when we have more information about their skills and needs.

Imagine being in a situation where someone underestimated your ability to do something. Perhaps someone assumed that because you were a woman you couldn't change a tire, or because you were a man you didn't know how to bake a cake, or perhaps because you were older you wouldn't know anything about computers when, in fact, you did? It would be incredibly frustrating, wouldn't it? Especially when they hadn't checked what you know or exactly what the problem is. They just assumed you didn't have the necessary knowledge or skill and proceeded to try to teach you something, or worse still, they didn't bother to explain something and just took over doing it themselves. Now, imagine if this was happening to you multiple times every day. How would you feel?

This is the experience that many neurodivergent children and adolescents have every day, especially when their different communication or learning styles make it more challenging for them to express their needs, or when myths about their neurotype lead to preconceived ideas about what they can and can't do. This illustrates why presuming competence is so important.

There are many powerful stories of non-speaking individuals who were unable to communicate and share their thoughts and feelings until someone in their life presumed competence and gave them the opportunities they needed to show their true selves. Some of these individuals have become advocates and share their stories in blogs and social media, some have become presenters at conferences and authors, and many more are now living their best lives at home, at school, and in the community. But none of this would be possible if someone had not seen their potential and offered them the tools they needed to succeed.

I would like to share a personal example of the power of presuming competence in our clients. Many years ago, I had the pleasure of working with a young girl called Kiah (I have received her permission to share her story) with cerebral palsy, epilepsy, and high support needs. She used a wheelchair for mobility, was non-speaking, and had very limited movement, but she was able to use her eyes to communicate with her mother and peers at preschool, and had a speech pathologist who had been active in finding effective ways for her to communicate using Augmentative and Alternate Communication (AAC). As a psychologist, I wanted to support Kiah with her transition to school, and her mother asked about assessing her cognitive function. At that time there was not a valid test that could be used for a child with such limited movement and communication, but we adapted the assessment materials of an IQ test to allow Kiah to respond with eye gaze so we could obtain an estimate of her skills. Her responses indicated she was at a similar level to her peers.

With this information, her mother was able to advocate for Kiah to be included in some mainstream learning and, with a supportive team behind her, to continue to learn to use more complex AAC and engage in the curriculum and other extra-curricular activities.

I was lucky enough to reconnect with Kiah in secondary school, and work with her and her team to continue to find ways for her to access learning and pursue her interests.

Now, at the age of 19, Kiah has just completed the first part of a bridging course to study at university, has a special interest in astrophysics, and is about to take part in her first youth summit to advocate for disability rights. Kiah has worked extremely hard to get to where she is now, and I am proud to say that I have been part of the team that has supported her to get there. And it all started from presuming competence.

In addition to acknowledging potential and providing opportunities that aren't limited by low expectations, there are some other ways we can show respect and presume competence with child and adolescent clients.

First, it is important that we don't talk down to or infantilize our clients. Even when language needs to be simplified to support a client's understanding, there is no need to speak to clients like they are babies. We need to just speak to them in a normal speaking voice. It is also important to have a range of activities and items available for children to use in therapy that reflect many different ages and interests. Don't assume that a teen client with an Intellectual Disability will not be interested in fashion magazines and pop culture just because they also still like baby dolls.

Second, it is essential that we don't talk about a child while they are present unless they are being included in the conversation. If you were attending a doctor to investigate a health concern, or had decided to see a psychologist to get some support with your mental health, would you expect to be part of the process? Or would you expect a partner or parent and the clinician to discuss your situation in front of you, without you having an opportunity to share information and ask questions? Unfortunately, it is all too common in the world of pediatrics, and especially with the disabled community, for children and adolescents to be spoken about while they are in the room like they are invisible.

Now, I am certainly aware that some children will not want to be involved in conversations about medical procedures, for example, and will be happy for a parent to be given that information, or perhaps would prefer that a parent give the clinician background information about an incident or concern. That is fine if it is the child's choice. However, even if a child is not directly engaging with you, it is important that they are acknowledged and given the opportunity to participate in the discussion regardless of whether they respond or not—after all, it is about them.

2. PROMOTE AUTONOMY

The issue of autonomy and consent is one that is contentious at the best of times, especially when it involves children and disability.

However, I believe it is something that needs to be discussed more openly and with consideration to giving children more autonomy in decisions about their lives and their bodies.

To be clear, I am not saying that all children will have the ability to make important decisions regarding their health and wellbeing, and obviously that is why parents are responsible for them. But what I am saying is that wherever possible we should be providing children with appropriate and accessible information that allows them to contribute to the therapeutic process.

One way to do this is to support a child or adolescent to give assent to participate in therapy. Rather than informed consent, which would be necessary for an adolescent or adult deemed to have the capacity to agree to a medical procedure with a full understanding of the risks and benefits, assent occurs when a child or adolescent agrees to be involved in a procedure or therapy following being provided with information adapted to their level of understanding. In this situation, their legal guardian takes on the burden of formal informed consent.

Ideally, this process should start before the clinician's first contact with a client. A client cannot give assent to participate in the therapeutic process if they do not know they are seeing a clinician and what they are seeing them for. Providing a parent with appropriate information for the child about who they are seeing and what might happen in a first session provides the child with an opportunity to understand where they are going and why. This may be as simple as a picture of the clinician and their description as a "special person who helps children" for a child with minimal ability to process the information, or a more detailed discussion about who the clinician is, what they do, and why a parent thinks seeing them will be beneficial for a child who can understand this kind of information. But it should not be assumed that a child does not need to be given any information due to their disability. As discussed earlier, it is important to *presume competence.*

While parents or professionals may feel that forcing a child to participate in therapy may be necessary and beneficial to the child, the reality is that forcing a child to do anything against their will can have a significant negative impact on their wellbeing as well as creating distrust in relationships.

Now this does not mean that a child who may be feeling unsure about something might not be willing to give it a try, or in the case of things such as chores may decide to push through discomfort to get some pocket money. But in these examples the child is making a choice to participate. This is different to a child being forced to do something when they don't feel safe, when they are feeling scared or anxious, or when it causes them pain.

If a child is frequently distressed about going to a regular appointment and doesn't want to attend, this is an indication that they do not assent to the therapy they are receiving, and other options may need to be considered.

Please note that I understand that a situation may arise when a child may need to be forced to do something when there is a serious or compelling reason, such as a situation that may seriously threaten a child or adult's safety, is a medical emergency, or would be considered at a similar level of urgency. But this should be a very rare occurrence.

Ultimately, if a child doesn't want to attend therapy, even after you, as the therapist, has adapted sessions to suit the child and get them involved, it may be best to cease service and refer them elsewhere, or consider providing support to a parent instead of the child. Any client who becomes distressed about attending and doesn't want to be in session is unlikely to get anything out of being there.

Once a child assents to participating in therapy or a medical appointment, clinicians should continue to provide opportunities for clients to be informed about what is happening in the session and that they can say "no" if they feel the need. This may be in the form of telling the child what you are doing (e.g., "I'm just going to look in your ear, it might feel cold") or having a visual schedule of activities planned for a session, but always with the possibility that the client may want to stop or say "no" at any time.

I am aware that for some health professionals and therapists, the idea of allowing a child to dictate what they will and won't do in a session may seem to go against more traditional views. Many of us have been brought up in environments where, by default, adults are in a position of authority, and as such should be obeyed. Especially in a therapy situation when the adult "knows what's best" for the child, it may seem counterintuitive to allow the child to have the "power" in a session. However, therapy should not be about control or power; it should be about collaboration and support. Further, we now know that a clinician who listens and adapts to their client's needs and stops when a child says "no" is a clinician a child is more likely to feel safe with over time, and as a result, will be able to participate with more.

Allowing a child to say "no" also helps to teach them that they have autonomy regarding their body and their actions, and that they have choices about what they do. It also helps them see that their feelings mean something and that there is power in their voice. Particularly for neurodivergent children who tend to spend a lot of their time being told to put others' needs before their own, learning that what they want is important and it is okay to put their own needs first is an important lesson that we can support them to learn. Being able to speak up and say "no" also gives rise to building confidence in self-advocacy, a skill that will have lifelong benefits.

As clinicians, working within a neurodiversity affirming framework and respecting a child's autonomy means it is our job to support our clients' needs, and to work towards their goals in ways that they feel safe and interested in, and are going to say "yes" to.

When a child engages with adults in ways that do not allow them to have a voice, and they are forced into compliance, they may learn that their wants and needs are not important, or worse, that they must comply with all adult direction without question, even when they feel unsafe or uncomfortable. This has the potential to set a child up to be more vulnerable to being groomed and abused, both as a child and in later life. Although this might sound extreme or far-fetched, reports of neurodivergent adults with lived experience of compliance-based therapies and settings support this premise.

Some individuals report experiences ranging from being extremely suggestible and easily led by others to situations in which they were taken advantage of or abused by people in positions of power, which they attribute, in some part, to their lack of autonomy and being trained to obey.

Overall, ensuring that we incorporate consent and assent into every part of our therapeutic approach provides children with the opportunity to maintain their autonomy and have choice and control in the therapeutic process, which creates a more positive and affirming experience.

3. RESPECT ALL COMMUNICATION STYLES

Being able to communicate clearly and consistently with a client is essential for any therapeutic relationship. However, in my experience clinicians do not receive enough training or support to practice in ways that cater to a variety of communication styles and formats.

When speech is your own primary mode of communication and the mode you are most comfortable working in, it can be daunting and feel well outside your comfort zone when you have a client who communicates in a different way. But it is important to remember that all communication is valid. When we take the time to get to know our clients, the way they communicate their wants and needs, and how they are best able to learn, we can be more effective clinicians and more affirming in our practice.

To be neurodiversity affirming with regard to communication, we need to be open to accepting and working with a variety of communication styles. If a child is non-speaking and uses body language to indicate their comfort or distress in sessions, perhaps by holding your hand and taking you to a particular activity in the room that they want to engage with, or squealing and pushing something away that they don't like, we need to acknowledge this as a real and valid way for them to communicate with us. We can use our own words to express what they are telling us (e.g., "You want to play with this now" or "You've finished playing with that" or "You're frustrated that it won't go together the way you wanted"). Then we can watch for indications in their facial expression and body language to ensure we have interpreted their communication correctly. If it seems like you have got it wrong, try again. Being understood is something that most of us take for granted, and it is important that we are showing our clients that we are invested in understanding and supporting them.

When a client is using AAC as their voice, it is essential that they have access to their materials or device throughout any therapy session, just as they would have access to their voice if they were speaking. The use of AAC may mean that the pace of a session is different and, if this is the case, clinicians need to adapt their expectations of what may be achieved in a session when there are time restraints, or factor in a client's fatigue when communicating. It is also important to resist the urge to jump in and finish a child's sentence for them or make assumptions about what they are going to say unless this is a system that has been agreed on together.

Another neurodivergent style of communication, particularly in Autistic children, is scripting. This is when a child uses set phrases or sentences to communicate, often ones that they have heard from other people or from favorite movies, books, or television shows. It is again important to recognize that even though this may not appear to be spontaneous language, it is still a valid way of communicating. In recent years this kind of language acquisition has been described as "Gestalt language processing" in which children learn and develop language through chunks or scripts of words that have a meaning, rather than learning and combining individual words. When working with a child who communicates in this way, it is important to consider the overall meaning of what they are saying rather than focusing on the individual words. In situations where a child is using specific sentences or phrases from movies or television shows, it can be particularly helpful to become familiar with the main sources of their language, as the context in which the language is used in the movie or television show may be relevant to the child's choice of phrase in their daily life.

But what about when a child can talk, but sometimes becomes mute and uses AAC or body language to communicate? Shouldn't we try and encourage them to talk when we know they can? The short answer to these questions is a resounding "NO." When we are accepting a child's communication efforts, whatever they are, we can't pick and choose how they communicate with us. There are many reasons why a child who can speak may be unable to at different times or in different situations, and even if it is just a preference or choice, it is their choice to make.

I have also found that for some children, particularly with the increase in the use of telehealth in recent years, communicating in writing such as by text message or in an online chat is sometimes preferred, and can provide an opportunity for discussions that would not be possible for the child in spoken word. It might even be writing on a notepad that is passed between you and the client. Ultimately it is about taking the child's lead and communicating in whatever format they are most comfortable with.

Now, we can't really have a discussion about neurodivergent communication without mentioning eye contact. Eye contact is a communication tool that is used by neurotypical individuals to connect, draw attention, and show interest in others. However, for many neurodivergent individuals, eye contact is avoided due to it feeling uncomfortable and not being a natural part of neurodivergent communication. Some neurodivergent individuals can and will use eye contact in certain situations, such as when they are talking about an interest or passion or to briefly catch someone's attention. Others may not use it at all. It is important to remember that as neurodiversity affirming clinicians, eye contact should never be forced when interacting with a client, and that we understand that a lack of eye contact does not mean that a child is not listening or paying attention to us or the situation they are in. In fact, for many neurodivergent individuals, it is easier to pay attention and process information when not making eye contact.

While we are being accepting of a child's communication style, whatever that may be, we also need to be mindful that we are communicating in a way that our clients can relate to. There is no point persisting with our usual way of communicating if it is not a modality that our clients are going to understand. This can be tricky, and is certainly very individual, as some clients will have much better receptive language skills than expressive skills (e.g., they could be non-speaking but have a good understanding of spoken language), and others may have well-developed expressive language but have challenges with understanding and processing the speech of others. Further still, some neurodivergent clients will find expression and understanding of language challenging and be more able to engage in interactions and process information if it is presented visually. As such, it is important that clinicians adapt their communication style to simplify language and incorporate visual prompts or AAC to support understanding for those clients who will benefit from this.

4. BE INFORMED BY NEURODIVERGENT VOICES

To truly understand the experience of all neurotypes and how to best support them in our work, it is essential that we listen to individuals with lived experience.

Just by virtue of the neurotypical neurotype being most prominent, there is an abundance of information about how neurotypical individuals experience everyday life. What they think and feel about their experiences, how they learn, process information, communicate and socialize, and how their needs can generally be catered for are accepted as common knowledge. However, this is not the case for the neurodivergent community.

Historically, the only information we had on the experience of different neurotypes was written by neurotypical researchers and clinicians, and was full of assumptions based on the latest theories and misconceptions about how disordered neurodivergent individuals were.

We now have access to a wide range of lived experience experts who can provide an insight into their specific neurotypes, share information on their strengths and challenges, and inform us as clinicians as to how we can better support them and the wider neurodivergent community.

I regularly come across professionals who are reluctant to listen to neurodivergent voices or who dismiss information gained from lived experience as being unscientific or not applicable to the wider neurodivergent community. What these professionals fail to recognize is that the reason we know so much about the neurotypical neurotype is that over hundreds of years neurotypical individuals have shared their knowledge and experiences. Researchers and clinicians have noticed patterns, questioned, theorized, and conducted research, and developed treatments and supports that have been created around this knowledge. So, listening to neurodivergent voices and being informed by them is the first step in developing further understanding and knowledge through research and clinical experience.

What is also often forgotten is that theories are usually based on what we know about something at one time. These theories evolve and change as we expand our knowledge and understanding. So it makes sense that with more information being available about the neurodivergent experience, theories about neurodivergence may change. This is what an evidence-based approach to therapy is all about. However, many professionals seem reluctant to accept that change (does anyone see the irony here?).

Neurodivergent adults were once children themselves, and so they have a wealth of knowledge and insights regarding their experience of growing up neurodivergent, what barriers they faced, and what supports were most helpful. Neurodivergent adults have given us an insight into the world of children who may not be able to share their innermost experiences. For example, there are a number of non-speaking adolescents and adults who use social media and blogging to share their experiences and advocate for the non-speaking members of their communities. This is invaluable information for anyone working with a neurodivergent child. It not only gives us an insight into the possible challenges of our clients; it also helps us understand and empathize, and ask the right questions to explore our client's experiences.

When we listen to neurodivergent voices, and use their experiences to inform our practice, we can do this from both a collective and an individual point of view. For example, there are many neurodivergent narratives that collectively demonstrate similar themes regarding the effectiveness of certain therapies, or challenges in the classroom or the workplace. These themes may not apply to everyone, but they are certainly worth taking into consideration with regard to clients and their needs, and exploring whether these broader ideas may be relevant to an individual client.

Then, from an individual point of view, we are informed by our clients in terms of their comfort, needs, and approaches to therapy, and whether the work we are doing with them is effective. We can gain this information in many ways, not just by the client telling us with words, and it is essential that we listen and adapt our practice to ensure we are supporting our clients and providing the best possible care.

Listening to neurodivergent individuals and incorporating their lived experience and knowledge into our practice is an essential part of being a neurodiversity affirming therapist, and, as already discussed, is necessary in order for us to be evidence-based in our practice.

5. TAKE A STRENGTHS-BASED APPROACH

Working in a strengths-based way is not a new concept in the therapeutic or clinical world. It is frequently used in approaches to support neurotypical individuals, and is also an integral part of trauma-informed practice (which we will discuss in the next chapter); however, its use with the disabled community is inconsistent, and this needs to change.

It may seem like focusing on strengths in therapy would be something that we are in the habit of doing, particularly when supporting children. However, going through a comprehensive assessment to identify neurodivergence usually involves highlighting deficits and impairments in relation to neurotypical development. Further, the process of applying for resources, public funding, and supports tends to be deficit-based. This negative bias in diagnostics and supports can then lead to an overall view of disability and neurodivergence as a bad thing. It can cloud the perspectives of parents and clinicians to only see the challenges a child will face.

Using a strengths-based approach is not about ignoring challenges; it is about recognizing that everyone has abilities and resources that can be used to help them achieve their goals. As neurodiversity affirming clinicians, we can work with our clients to identify and build on the skills and supports they already have, and focus on what they can do now and want to do in the future rather than getting stuck on what they can't do.

A strengths-based approach not only considers an individual's personal strengths, but also how conditions in their environment can be adapted to remove barriers and facilitate access to desired activities. This is in keeping with the social model of disability. It is about identifying what a neurodivergent individual wants to do, and looking at what adaptations and accommodations need to be made to allow that individual to have access to their desired activity. For example, in the case of a Dyslexic child who wants to write a children's book, we could provide access to speech-to-text software to support the child to record their story in writing, assist them to divide the text into pages based on what content they want included, and give them access to art materials or software to draw the illustrations. Just because they have difficulty with reading and spelling doesn't mean that writing a book has to be out of reach for them.

Individuals may also have access to family, friends, and members of the community who are part of their team and can act as resources to support an individual to achieve. For example, if a teen in a wheelchair wanted to go to the beach, we would need to consider how to transport them there, and then how to support them to access the beach itself. This may require choosing a beach that has accessible ramps already installed, a wheelchair-accessible vehicle to get them there, and a support person to accompany them across the beach to the water. With planning and resources, any barriers can be managed so that individuals have opportunities instead of limits.

Working in a strengths-based way is about being open to possibilities, being curious about how something can be done even if it seems unlikely, and utilizing a child's personal strengths and other resources to make things happen.

6. HONOR NEURODIVERGENT CULTURE

As we have already discussed, being neurodiversity affirming means seeing neurodivergent neurotypes as different from the norm rather than impaired. This gives rise to the notion that neurodivergence can be viewed as its own culture, one characterized by differences in communication, sensory sensitivities, cognition, and behaviors.

Now, a discussion could certainly be had regarding whether each neurodivergent neurotype should be seen as its own culture. But for the purposes of this section, I would like to consider neurodivergent neurotypes as a collective whole, which to me makes sense given the substantial overlap between many neurodivergent characteristics across neurotypes.

Honoring neurodivergent culture is about accepting neurodivergent individuals for who they are and not trying to change them to make them appear more "normal."

Unfortunately, from a historical perspective that is exactly what therapy for neurodivergent individuals has been about—trying to take away any obvious signs of neurodivergence to make them fit in with neurotypical society.

In therapy, we can honor our clients' neurodivergence by giving them a safe space to be themselves, accommodating their needs, and being accepting of their neurodivergent style of being. This means that clinicians may need to adapt the environment in which they see clients to support sensory sensitivities (e.g., dimming the lights, having a tent to retreat to, providing fidget toys, etc.), and be open and flexible in how they conduct their sessions and interact with their clients to accommodate neurodivergent communication and learning.

This may look like a client being free to engage in stimming openly when needed, or to spend time info-dumping about their favorite television show or the qualities of their favorite fungi. It could be providing space for a child to pace around the room or play with fidget toys while talking, or to work on the floor or under the desk or in the hallway to complete activities. A clinician might use videos to support understanding of concepts rather than books or written materials, or incorporate a child's interests into sessions to support attention and focus. Or perhaps a client will play or create art to express themselves and process their experiences, and not talk at all. Each client's expression of neurodivergent culture will be specific to the individual and needs to be recognized and accommodated rather than becoming a focus for change in therapy.

When neurodivergent characteristics such as "black and white thinking" or "stimming" or being "sensory-seeking" or "not making eye contact" are highlighted as problems in thinking or behavior that need to be changed, this sends the message to neurodivergent children that they are faulty or broken, and that they need to change who they are to be accepted. Therapies that focus on changing these qualities more often than not lead to masking in the individual, and rather than improving the client's life, result in poor self-esteem and self-worth, and poorer mental health outcomes.

This does not mean that an individual may not benefit from support to engage in problem-solving techniques that help them see the "gray" in situations, or to understand the way neurotypical people communicate, but it needs to be done in a way that does not pathologize their natural way of being.

Ironically, there are qualities attributed to neurodivergent individuals (e.g., rigid or inflexible thinking) that are also found in the neurotypical population and contribute to the neurodivergent community's difficulties. As one of my teen clients often says, "neurotypical people say we are inflexible, but they don't see that we are having to change the way we do things every day to fit in with them because they won't change."

Honoring our clients' neurodivergent culture and giving them the message that they are accepted and valued just as they are is an important part of neurodiversity affirming practice, and can make a big difference to how our clients see themselves.

7. TAILOR SUPPORTS TO INDIVIDUAL NEEDS

When we talk about tailoring an approach specifically to a client's needs, this not only means adapting our communication and the way we present information; it is also about recognizing neurodivergent experience as different to the neurotypical perspective, and ensuring that we honor our client's experiences throughout this process.

Due to differences in sensory processing, cognition, communication, and perception, neurodivergent individuals experience the world differently to the neurotypical population, and as such are likely to present in therapy with different challenges or to have different underlying needs.

This can be demonstrated through our understanding of anxiety in Autistic individuals. Recent research has found that Autistic individuals can experience anxiety similarly to neurotypical individuals, with unhelpful cognitions and physiological symptoms. But they can also experience Autistic-specific anxiety, which has different qualities, such as having no associated unhelpful cognitions or having a purely sensory trigger. If we were to approach an Autistic individual's anxiety only in ways designed for the neurotypical population, we may completely miss the underlying cause and be suggesting supports or strategies to assist that will ultimately not be effective.

An example of this is a teen client I see who presents with anxiety and specific phobia. There were clear cognitions she could identify around some of her anxiety triggers, and others that were more sensory in nature; however, she was still experiencing anxiety-like symptoms, such as increased heart rate, dizziness, and rapid breathing, in the absence of any obvious cause. She was fed up with therapists telling her to think certain things or do deep breathing in these moments because neither of these strategies was effective, and she was made to feel she wasn't doing it right or working hard enough to manage these challenges. Following some investigations by her doctor and specialist testing, it was found that she has Postural Orthostatic Tachycardia syndrome (POTS) and blood pressure irregularities that were causing these episodes—it was nothing to do with her cognitions or sensory sensitivities, and was best managed with medication and rest.

Further, a recent research study conducted in the UK with Autistic adults found that one of the biggest barriers to therapy being effective was that it was not tailored to the client's individual needs. This included accessibility to therapy itself (e.g., home-based, telehealth, or clinic-based, etc.), and the modalities in which therapy was undertaken.

While the client may not know what kind of approach is going to work best, they often do know what communication style is most effective for them to take in information (e.g., written, oral, video, etc.) and what they need to feel most comfortable in a therapy setting (e.g., sensory preferences such as lighting, noise, movement), and these are things we can ask about right at the start of our relationship and take into consideration for our sessions.

Then we can work with a client to understand their individual experiences and try different approaches or a combination of therapeutic modalities to find what is going to suit them best.

Chapter 5

Which Therapy Approaches Are Considered Neurodiversity Affirming?

You may already suspect from what you now know of neurodiversity affirming practice that the idea of neurodiversity affirming therapy approaches is not straightforward. While there are some therapy approaches that are considered more affirming than others, it is also the way the therapist engages in the approach that is important in determining whether it is considered neurodiversity affirming.

Even though some readers may be from professions that do not provide therapy themselves, it is good to be educated on what to look for in a therapeutic approach and in a therapist to assist children and families to make educated choices about their supports.

It is important to note that at the time of writing this book (2023) there was limited research available on effective therapies for neurodivergent individuals that were affirming in their design and approach. Further, of the research that was available, most of it was focused on adult participants and therapies, and as such, we continue to have little concrete data about how best to support neurodivergent children and adolescents.

Fortunately, what we do have are neurodivergent adults who have been willing to share their experience of different therapies in childhood. We also have children and adolescents who are now being empowered to share their experiences and inform clinicians about what works and what doesn't, and therapist allies who listen to these voices, and incorporate their training and expertise with lived experience to achieve the best possible outcomes for their neurodivergent clients.

Before a child is even referred for therapeutic supports, if we are being truly neurodiversity affirming, the first question to ask is "Does the child need therapy?" Just because a child is neurodivergent doesn't mean they will need therapy. There are certainly many reasons why therapy could be helpful for a neurodivergent child, and these may include challenges they are facing due to their neurodivergence, health conditions that cause pain or distress, or perhaps stress and trauma caused by other people and their environment. But a child should not be put in therapy just because they are different.

Once we have established whether engaging in therapy will be appropriate and useful, we then need to think about what is involved in the therapy itself.

WHAT DOES NEURODIVERSITY AFFIRMING THERAPY LOOK LIKE?

First, neurodiversity affirming therapy should be driven by the principles described in Chapter 4 in that it: presumes competence; promotes autonomy; respects all communication styles; is informed by neurodivergent voices; is strengths-based; honors neurodivergent culture; and is tailored to the individual's needs.

In practice, with these principles in mind, once we have established that there is a benefit to accessing therapy and that the individual is not being pushed to conform to neurotypical ways of thinking and feeling, the next step is to listen to the client's experience of their challenges, develop an understanding of how they work best, and then explore possible approaches with the client to find a good fit. This doesn't mean that once you decide on an approach that you must only use that one modality to support the individual, but it gives you a starting point. Then you can adapt and collaborate as you go along depending on what appears to be effective and what doesn't, as you tailor the approach specifically to your client and their individual needs.

This will involve incorporating your client's preferred communication style into sessions, providing information and resources in formats that are accessible to your client, working in more direct or indirect ways depending on your client's needs, and adapting to the changing therapeutic environment. It is good to note that therapeutic approaches that are extremely prescriptive and follow a very specific structure that can't be deviated from are unlikely to be neurodiversity affirming, as there needs to be flexibility for clients to choose what they share, how fast they go, and how they participate.

Generally speaking, trauma-informed approaches are often considered neurodiversity affirming due to their focus on individual needs and their acknowledgment of the impact that experiences have on our brains and bodies, and how we perceive the world. These approaches highlight the need for physical and psychological safety and trusting relationships in the therapeutic space, and recognize that without these factors, therapy is not going to be successful.

Trauma-informed approaches also promote acceptance of all emotions and responses as valid and real for the individual, and treat them accordingly. This means that an individual will not have their emotions or perceptions dismissed by a therapist in favor of the "right" response to a situation.

However, even within trauma-informed therapies, there are elements that may not fit with neurodiversity affirming principles. For example, exposure therapy is often used as part of trauma-informed therapy programs to desensitize individuals to triggering situations so that over time they can participate in activities without being impacted greatly by their past traumatic experiences. While this may be appropriate for some neurotypical individuals, research suggests that neurodivergent individuals do not easily become desensitized to environments, especially when there is sensory sensitivity involved. This means that rather than growing accustomed to a situation or stimulus, neurodivergent individuals may instead be re-traumatized by being exposed to triggering situations repeatedly as part of graded exposure.

Approaches such as Cognitive Behavior Therapy have also been criticized at times for supporting the idea of "thinking errors" that must be corrected, which could be interpreted as promoting the notion that there are correct and incorrect ways of thinking. This is particularly problematic when the "errors" identified are naturally part of neurodivergent thinking patterns. We can avoid this, however, by not focusing on overall thinking patterns, and instead identifying the distressing thoughts specifically, and targeting those thoughts in therapy.

So, while there are many therapeutic approaches that can be made to be neurodiversity affirming if clinicians are aware and adapt their practice accordingly, there are also some approaches that are widely seen as being more affirming than others. These approaches include Dialectical Behavior Therapy, Eye Movement Desensitization and Reprocessing, Acceptance and Commitment Therapy, Child-Centered Play Therapy, Creative Arts Therapy, and Animal-Assisted Therapy.

There are also a number of neurodivergent professionals who are adapting therapeutic approaches specifically for neurodivergent populations and sharing their methods in books and training, which is providing clinicians with more specific guidance on how to use these approaches in neurodiversity affirming ways. This is a fantastic opportunity to learn from individuals with both clinical knowledge and lived experience.

Ultimately, being neurodiversity affirming in practice is up to us as clinicians and the choices we make in how we support our clients. In the coming chapters in Parts 2 and 3 we will explore some specific ways that we can be neurodiversity affirming when supporting clients with some common reasons for seeking therapy.

A NOTE ABOUT BEHAVIORAL THERAPIES

Content Warning: Behavioral therapies, Applied Behavior Analysis (ABA), trauma.

There has been much discussion in recent years about the use of therapies such as Applied Behavior Analysis (ABA), Early Intensive Behavioral Intervention, and others that have their roots in behaviorism. While these therapies have been traditionally focused on Autistic children, more general behavioral approaches have been used with other children with disabilities and also with the neurotypical population for many years, albeit less intensely.

ABA has been around for decades and has, for much of that time, been considered the "gold standard" therapy for Autistic children. In its early years it was primarily focused on reducing Autistic behaviors in children, such as stimming, and training children to comply with adult direction and to carry out specific learning tasks through positive reinforcement and punishment, with children recommended to be receiving at least 20 hours of ABA every week. While proponents of modern ABA say that it has changed and is now more flexible and naturalistic, it is still entrenched in behavioral theory, and involves repetitive transactional interactions that are reinforced by the therapist for hours and hours every week, usually at a high financial cost to families.

One of the biggest concerns that critics of ABA have is that it takes away a child's autonomy by forcing compliance and not acknowledging or meeting a child's social-emotional or sensory needs. Many autistic adults who were put through ABA as children report being traumatized by the experience, having had their discomfort and distress ignored, and being forced to comply with their behavior therapist's instruction to avoid punishment or endless repetitions of the same questions and responses.

While ABA and its other forms has been widely researched within its own ranks and found to be effective in supporting Autistic children, most of this research has not held up to scrutiny. In fact, recent independent research conducted by large organizations such as the US Department of Defense have found that ABA is not effective in providing positive outcomes for Autistic children. Research also now suggests that more hours of therapy are not associated with better outcomes, bringing the cost and intensity of ABA programs into question.

Strict behavioral therapies such as ABA do not have a place in neurodiversity affirming practice. If you would like to know more about this topic, please see the "Useful Resources" section for some Autistic-led resources and information.

— PART 2 —

IN PRINCIPLE

In this second part of the book, I would like to take you through some important considerations in working with all clients, but particularly with the neurodivergent community. As I have previously mentioned, there are common elements of any therapeutic process that are routinely completed with neurotypical clients but frequently glossed over or ignored completely with the neurodivergent population. I wanted to bring these important elements to your attention to help you reflect on your own practice, and to explore whether there is room for you to be more neurodiversity affirming with your clients.

— Chapter 6 —

The Therapeutic Relationship

The therapeutic relationship is one of the strongest predictors of positive outcomes in therapy, according to research. However, in my experience it receives minimal focus in clinician training, often only being discussed as necessary to "build rapport" in a client's first session. Then there is an expectation that children will move straight into "therapy."

It may, in fact, be the case that neurotypical children who have had mostly positive experiences with adults in their past will respond to this approach. However, neurotypical children are not likely to be bombarded with new sensory information that is threatening to overwhelm them, and probably find it easy to generalize the experiences from other medical appointments and therapy sessions they have had. So it is easier for them to feel safe, develop a sense of trust, and quickly fall into a familiar "teacher–student" type relationship where the adult tells you what to do and you do it.

However, for the majority of neurodivergent children, experience with adults will likely have been varied and inconsistent. And experiences in medical settings and therapy rooms may have been tolerable at best, and distressing at worst, unless they have been lucky enough to have found a clinician who really understands them.

While you may think it is an exaggeration to say that neurodivergent children will have much more challenging experiences with adults than their neurotypical peers, consider how often neurodivergent children are likely to be criticized or reprimanded for their behavior when it does not fit neurotypical expectations (e.g., stimming, impulsiveness, emotional regulation challenges, sensory sensitivities, being disrespectful or rude, not trying hard enough, etc.), particularly when outside the home. For example, it has been estimated by psychiatrist Dr. William W. Dodson that, by the age of 12, ADHDers have received 20,000 more negative messages from parents, teachers, and other adults than their same aged peers (Dodson 2016).

So, developing a therapeutic relationship with your neurodivergent client, in which they feel safe, secure, and able to trust, may not be an easy thing to do.

Given that a key element of neurodiversity affirming practice is acceptance, it makes sense that the concept of "unconditional positive regard" should be important in therapeutic relationships with neurodivergent children. Unconditional positive regard (UPR) is a concept first introduced by psychologist Carl Rogers as part of his humanistic and client-centered approach to therapy (see Farber, Suzuki, and Ort 2022). UPR is about accepting an individual fully for who they are without judgment, regardless of what they say or do. It means seeing past a child's challenges and behaviors to the child underneath, and finding a genuine connection.

All children want to be liked and accepted, but many have developed pictures of themselves as unlovable or as failures, and will find it hard to connect with adults because they don't think they deserve love and support. Other children may have been let down or criticized so much by adults that they don't feel safe or that they can trust anyone.

Showing your client that you genuinely accept, like, and care about them can take a considerable amount of time and effort with children who have had these negative experiences in their history. Some clients will test you to see if you really do care, but it is absolutely worth it. For example, I have found that taking time to develop some knowledge and understanding about one of your client's interests can be one way to demonstrate your care and interest in connecting with them. You may think that a child should be fine with you because you don't have history with them, but a child's early experiences can have lasting effects, and it takes a long time for a child to heal. Ultimately, consistently responding with care and curiosity regardless of the child's actions, and not taking their behavior personally, will help them see that you really do accept them and understand that they are doing as well as they can.

Also remember that children are generally very intuitive to the attitude of adults, so they will know if you don't genuinely care for them and may act out as a result. Even though some clients may be hard to get to know at the start, usually with persistence and openness you will be able to find a way to connect and see their endearing side. If you are having difficulty giving a child UPR and accepting them for who they are, seeking supervision from a senior clinician can be a helpful way to explore why this is the case, and to support you to make changes to repair or improve your relationship with the child. If this is not possible, it may be necessary to refer the child on to someone who can better meet their needs.

I should clarify here that unconditional acceptance does not equal no boundaries. However, it does mean that a child is not punished or shamed if they say or do something that falls outside what is acceptable within your practice. Instead, it is about acknowledging their feelings or heightened arousal, and deciding to take a break or perhaps cease a session and start afresh next time. The child needs to know that no matter what they do or what mistakes they might make, you are there for them.

Another important element to neurodiversity affirming practice and relationship-building is attunement. Attunement can be described as being deeply tuned into a client's thoughts and feelings. This allows us to better read and understand a client's emotions and experiences, and to empathize with them. To be truly attuned, we must be able to understand the experience of our clients and find a way to relate to them. When working with neurodivergent children, this means putting aside preconceived neurotypical notions of what their experiences might be, and really listening to their point of view.

Even as a multiply neurodivergent clinician myself, I find it helpful to listen to the lived experience of other neurodivergent adults and children, to broaden my understanding of what my clients may have experienced and how they may be feeling, because we are, of course, all different. It is also essential to be fully present with your clients in session, really focusing on not just what they say, but how their arousal levels might change and how they express their emotions, so you can reflect this and let them know you understand. For non-speaking clients, we can really attend to their non-verbal communication in session, and again monitor things like the child's arousal level to get an idea of how they might be feeling and what they need. When I talk about reflections, I am talking about those moments where we might comment on how we think a client is feeling in the moment, or perhaps how they felt or what they thought during an experience they are recounting, as a way of letting the child know we hear them and understand.

Generally speaking, if you mostly get your reflections of a child's thoughts and feelings right, they will be comfortable correcting you when you occasionally make a mistake. If you find yourself constantly getting it wrong and your client doesn't relate to how you are interpreting their experiences, you may need to take a step back and assess what you are missing in your interactions.

Regarding showing empathy, some neurodivergent individuals, and in particular Autistics, will recount a similar experience of their own to show that they understand and care about their friend's experience. This can often be misinterpreted by neurotypical individuals as them trying to get attention when it is, in fact, a way to show they care. I have found that many of my neurodivergent clients respond well to hearing about my own or other children's similar experiences to assist them to process what has happened to them, and to find comfort in knowing that they are not alone in feeling that way. This can be another way of connecting with a client and showing them you care.

A final essential element in relationship-building with clients is trust. When you think about the nature of medical and allied health, we are often seeing children at their most vulnerable. They are coming to us because they are sick or injured, distressed, or struggling, and need help. We expect them to be open and honest with us about their challenges and feelings, and in the case of medical professionals, to allow us to touch and examine their bodies, and we often see them at their worst. It makes sense then that we should take time to show that we can be trusted, and that we will indeed do what we say and do our best to help them in whatever capacity we can.

Our clients need to feel safe in our presence and trust that we won't do anything to harm or upset them. One way we can establish trust is by being consistent and predictable in our behavior and response to our clients. They need to know that each time they come to see us, we will interact with them in the same way. If we are calm and accepting of them one week, and then are irritated or angry with them the next, they will likely feel uncertain and uncomfortable about seeing us again because we have shown ourselves to be unpredictable.

Another important factor in developing trust is being honest. If a clinician makes promises they don't keep, or says they will do something and then don't do it, this will build mistrust. Similarly, if they lie to clients, perhaps with the intention of making something easier or less distressing, children will often pick up on this and know there is something wrong or untrustworthy about the clinician. Clients need to know that when you tell them something, it is the truth, even if it is difficult to hear.

When a child is able to trust you, they will feel confident that you will not do anything to harm them, and in turn are likely to be able to try new things or do things they may feel a bit nervous about because they know that you will not ask them to do anything dangerous or that they are not capable of doing.

With a strong relationship, we can support our clients to learn and develop in ways that will make a positive difference to their lives.

— Chapter 7 —

Goal-Setting

Collaborating with clients to support them to achieve their desired outcomes in therapy is an essential part of neurodiversity affirming practice. Setting goals can be important, not just to have a clear direction and focus for therapy, but also to meet the necessary requirements of most funding bodies providing supports and services. However, the way goals are written and what aims therapy seeks to achieve are important considerations in ensuring we are working in a neurodiversity affirming way to support our clients.

One of the biggest mistakes I see when working with neurodivergent children is that parents, educators, and service providers often create goals based just on what they want the child to do or stop doing—things that might make their lives easier because the child will be more compliant, or reduce behavior they see as challenging, or help the child to be more independent and take responsibility for their actions. While the outcomes might be beneficial for the child, they are looking at things from the wrong direction. Instead of thinking about what the child needs to learn or change in order to make things easier for others, we need to be considering what the child can learn or change to reduce distress and improve the child's quality of life, and what the adults in the child's life can do to support the child to make that happen.

Something that we need to be mindful of when we are talking about improving a child's life is our perception of quality of life and what it means to be successful. It is important that clinicians do not assume that what we or society may think is important in life equates to what an individual wants or values. For example, Dr. Peter Vermeulen, a counselor, educator, and researcher well known for his work with Autistic individuals, has created measures for Autistic quality of life and has described differences in wellbeing and success as defined by the Autistic community (see the "Useful Resources" at the end of the book for links to his work). It is important that, as professionals in an individual's life, we support them to develop skills and achieve what is important to them.

When working with children, it is often the case that goals are set for therapy without consultation with the child. While many children will not be able to directly contribute to goal-setting, they are often able to indicate aspects of their life that they would like to be easier or better, and these things can be incorporated into therapy goals. This is important because if a child has some ownership of what they are working on or want to achieve, and the goals are meaningful to them, they are much more likely to participate fully and, in turn, see better outcomes.

I do recognize that for some individuals, their ability to share their wants and needs may be limited, and at these times it is about the individual's parents supporting them to communicate, or perhaps communicating for them if necessary. However, the focus should still be the individual and what will make their life easier and better. Even when a child cannot indicate what they want to work on in therapy, it is important that goals are set from the child's point of view.

Unfortunately, it is still common to see goals in therapy and support plans—such as "Johnny will listen and comply with adult instructions in class" or "Sally will learn to react appropriately to challenges in her environment"—that focus on unrealistic expectations of children and are not really in the child's best interests. As clinicians, we need to support families and children to create meaningful and functional goals that are affirming in their wording and in the execution of therapy.

When considering whether a goal is affirming or not, the first thing to think about is how it is going to benefit the child. Is the goal trying to make the child more normal? Is it about making life easier for them and perhaps supporting skill development, or is it about making them conform and comply with adult direction and expectations? Any goals that aim to reduce neurodivergent characteristics that do not cause a child any difficulty or distress (e.g., stimming, info-dumping, special interests, sensory needs) would not be considered neurodiversity affirming. Goals that take away a child's autonomy and ignore their social-emotional and developmental needs would also not be considered affirming. For example, goals such as "Thomas will have quiet hands and sit cross-legged on the mat for story time" or "Milly will stay calm and not get upset when finishing her turn on the computer" do not respect the child's sensory or emotional needs, and place the responsibility of achieving these goals solely on the child.

Let's take the goal of "Thomas will have quiet hands and sit cross-legged on the mat for story time" as an example. To begin with, what is the purpose of this goal, and how will it benefit the child? Does Thomas even like story time? If the purpose is for Thomas to sit still and not be disruptive, this is not affirming. If the purpose is to teach Thomas how to sit cross-legged and not move his hands or touch others, this is also not affirming. If Thomas loves books and listening to stories but becomes dysregulated when sitting still to listen, and being dysregulated results in him being moved away and missing the story, then the purpose of the goal should be to help Thomas to be regulated during story time, which is affirming. However, the way the goal has been written doesn't reflect this or what his needs may be. If we determine that Thomas needs movement to regulate, and that it can be difficult for him to concentrate and focus his attention on the story being read without this accommodation, his goal needs to incorporate this. A more affirming goal might be "Thomas will be supported to listen to a book at story time with various seating options, space to move safely, and sensory tools to assist him to regulate." This goal is affirming because it identifies the activity Thomas wants to be involved in, acknowledges Thomas's needs, mentions the accommodations that are required, and recognizes that Thomas needs support rather than being expected to achieve this goal himself.

Another important factor to consider is whether the goals are appropriate for the child's developmental level and overall ability. It is often the case that parents and educators want a child to be able to complete tasks that are not realistic due to their disability, and may inadvertently set up a child to fail. Particularly for young children, expectations for skills and behavior that a child can complete independently are often overestimated, and the need for adults to support the child is often overlooked. For example, I often see goals for young ADHDers that relate to being more focused and reducing impulsivity. In the neurotypical population, executive functioning skills do not really start to become evident until around seven years of age and continue to develop into early adulthood. Is it reasonable, then, to expect that a five-year-old ADHDer is going to be able to quickly develop the skills needed to focus better and be less impulsive? Probably not. Instead, there needs to be an acknowledgment of their developing brain, the areas that are challenging, and what the adults around them can do to support them to be more focused and less impulsive, rather than the burden being on the child to change when they are developmentally not yet ready.

In some cases, it may be possible for clinicians to support parents to understand the skills a child may need to develop first before they can achieve the suggested goal, and adjust therapy goals accordingly to reflect the smaller steps needed to work towards a more long-term goal. In other cases, it may be necessary to focus more on how to assist the child to carry out challenging tasks until they are developmentally able to learn the necessary skills, and to educate parents on why the goal is not appropriate at the current time.

Whether the child has the capacity to engage and benefit from the therapeutic process is another factor in formulating goals. While skill development in a particular area such as emotional regulation may be beneficial for the child, they may still be too young to actually use their knowledge or strategies independently to effectively manage their emotions in different situations, and as such they may be reliant on co-regulation by a parent or adult and accommodations being made in the environment to actually be able to achieve the goal that has been set. If this is the case, working with the parents instead of directly with the child can be the most effective way to support the child and family, and goals should reflect this.

Being neurodiversity affirming with goal-setting is about collaborating with clients and families to create meaningful and functional goals that focus on what the client wants and needs. Goals should acknowledge the skills a child brings with them, and build on these to support them to achieve success in developing new skills and participating in new experiences while identifying supports and accommodations that may be beneficial so that the responsibility to make changes isn't always just on them. Working together with clients with a neurodiversity affirming approach, clinicians can ensure that therapy focuses on meaningful outcomes that clients are invested in reaching, with their support.

— Chapter 8 —

Sensory Differences and Regulation

Our sensory system is one of the main sources of information for our brain and body to adapt to our environment and regulate our arousal level. It is now widely accepted that there are eight senses that impact on our experience of the world. These eight sensory systems in simple terms are Vision, Hearing, Smell, Taste, Touch, Vestibular, Proprioceptive, and Interoceptive.

Differences in sensory processing are evident in the general population but appear to be more prominent in neurodivergent individuals. While sensory sensitivities are most commonly associated with being Autistic and are included in the official diagnostic criteria, other neurodivergent populations such as ADHDers and Dyslexics have also been shown to experience significant differences in sensory processing.

Given the higher frequency of sensory differences in neurodivergent individuals, it is an important part of neurodiversity affirming practice to acknowledge and accommodate individual sensory preferences and sensitivities to not only support clients to feel safe and comfortable in clinical settings, but also to recognize the impact of sensory processing differences on an individual's quality of life.

Neurodivergent individuals tend to experience either low or high thresholds to sensory input that can vary between sensory modalities.

Having a high threshold to sensory input means having a brain that doesn't recognize and process all the sensory information that is coming in, so it tends to miss a lot of sensory cues. Conversely, having a low threshold means having a brain that is extremely sensitive to sensory information, and as such tends to become easily overloaded by sensory input. Many neurodivergent brains also do not habituate, or get used, to sensory stimulation over time, meaning that repeated exposure to a sensory environment in order to make a child "get used to it" will not work.

Neurodivergent brains are also often saturated by sensory input, making it difficult to block out or filter distracting or distressing sensory information. For example, while a neurotypical individual might notice that there is someone talking quietly outside their classroom and then tune the noise out to focus on a lesson, a neurodivergent child might have difficulty listening to their teacher due to the noise outside.

One of the biggest issues I see regarding sensory sensitivities in children is the tendency for adults to respond to a child's sensory experience by saying that a noise "isn't that loud" or a touch "wasn't too hard," and dismissing their discomfort or distress as an overreaction. In reality, due to differing sensory systems, something that might feel like a small bump to one person could be painful to another, and as such an individual's sensory experience should be acknowledged and validated rather than diminished or ignored.

In contrast to children with low sensory thresholds, children who have a high threshold to sensory input may seek out sensory stimulation in the form of seeking movement or vestibular input (e.g., wriggling in their seat, getting up and moving around, rocking on a chair, rolling on the floor), resulting in them being reprimanded for not being focused and sitting still to complete activities.

Other children may be labeled as too rough, clumsy, or careless, and not knowing their own strength when they inadvertently hurt peers while playing, or they constantly bump into things and fall over, when really these children might just have poor proprioception and don't easily sense where their body is in space.

These are all important things to consider in clinical spaces because, for example, a child may find physical examination painful due to sensitivities to touch, or be easily over-extended and injured in physical therapy due to not being aware of their body's limits. Checking in with your client and listening to them when they say they are in pain or are finding sensory stimulation uncomfortable is important and can assist with providing the most affirming supports.

With regard to making the overall clinical environment more affirming and accommodating of sensory needs, there are some simple things we can put in place. It is easier to reduce the sensory impact of an environment and then provide sensory stimulation to someone who needs it, rather than having an environment that is going to bombard any client with sensory stimuli that may be uncomfortable. For example, having lights that can be dimmed or covers over fluorescent lighting to reduce the glare can make a big difference to clients who are sensitive to light or find visual stimulation difficult or painful. When these options aren't available, allowing clients to wear caps or tinted glasses to reduce visual input can be equally as accommodating.

For clients who need more sensory stimulation to feel comfortable, providing visually stimulating objects such as visual timers, having fidget toys and different textures to touch, or even having some of a client's favorite music playing, and allowing different seating or allowing them to move around the room can all make a difference.

AROUSAL AND REGULATION

Sensory-processing differences also contribute to an individual's arousal level at any point in time. When we talk about arousal, we are talking about how alert we are in any given situation. Arousal is associated with attention and focus and having the appropriate level of energy to engage in and complete tasks.

Our arousal level fluctuates throughout the day, and so can sensory sensitivities, which can then impact on an individual's ability to regulate their arousal level. Regulation is our ability to change and maintain our arousal level according to the needs of a task or the environment we are in to perform optimally. It is important to note here that being regulated does not just mean being calm. Being regulated means being in the right arousal state to carry out a certain activity. For example, if I am about to run a race, being calm won't assist me to perform at an optimal level. Instead, I need to be extra alert and energized to perform at my best when the starter's gun fires.

When a child's sensory system detects and/or processes information in different ways, it may be difficult for them to remain regulated in certain situations, impacting on their ability to participate in activities and learn. With neurodivergent sensory systems constantly taking in and processing sensory information without an effective filter, it is easy to see how many neurodivergent children may become dysregulated.

To help with understanding the importance of regulation to a child's ability to function in different environments, and particularly in clinical settings, I refer to the work of Dr. Bruce Perry, a world renowned psychiatrist who created the Neurosequential Model of Therapeutics and is known for his groundbreaking work on developmental trauma. Dr. Perry is an expert on early brain development and the neuroscience of relational safety, and created the 3 Rs (Regulate, Relate, Reason) to assist with understanding how regulation and connection support children to move from processing information in the "survival" parts of their brain to processing information using their "thinking brain" or cortex. Without support to regulate, which we can provide through safe sensory stimuli, children are unable to connect with us to feel safe and are not able to shift into an arousal state that will allow them to think and learn.

It is essential that as clinicians we recognize and incorporate sensory needs into our clinical environments and our sessions to support children to be regulated and to be able to engage in the therapeutic process, whether that is to learn about feelings, practice speech sounds, develop handwriting skills, or participate in a medical examination.

A NOTE ABOUT STIMMING

Stimming, or self-stimulatory behavior, can be described as a repetitive movement, use of an object, or activity that often involves a sensory aspect (e.g., hand flapping, rocking, spinning, humming, flicking a rubber band, listening to a song repeatedly, watching the credits of movies repeatedly, etc.). Stimming is once again something that does occur in the general population but is more common in neurodivergent individuals, and particularly in the Autistic community.

Unfortunately, stimming has historically been a big focus of behavior change in neurodivergent individuals due to it often being viewed as abnormal or disruptive and needing to be stopped so a child (or adult) will appear more "normal."

We now know that stimming serves a number of important purposes including enjoyment or pleasure, arousal regulation (often through increasing or decreasing sensory input), and management of stress and anxiety.

Being neurodiversity affirming means that we accept features of neurodivergence without trying to change them, and stimming is no exception. As such, a child should not be prevented from stimming unless it is causing harm to the child or someone else (e.g., self-injurious behavior).

When a child stims for pleasure or enjoyment, their stim may not be available to them all the time, or might not be possible to engage in whenever they want due to constraints of the environment. If this is the case, their stim should be available to them when possible, to allow them to engage in something they enjoy and take comfort in, just as neurotypical individuals engage in enjoyable activities. The opportunity to engage in stimming should never be contingent on behavior or used as a reward.

In situations where a child uses stimming to regulate their arousal or emotions, this is actually an adaptive skill that can be very effective and should be allowed unless it is harmful. If there are environmental factors that are likely to be causing a child distress or making it difficult for them to regulate, resulting in the child needing to stim, then making changes to the environment so the child feels more safe, secure, and regulated may remove their need to stim for this reason and allow them to engage more in activities around them that are of interest.

Even in a situation where a stim may be causing harm, it is important to determine what purpose the stim serves for the child, and explore whether environmental changes need to be implemented or a safer replacement can be found that can provide the child with the sensory input they need without causing injury.

— Chapter 9 —

Reframing Behavior

Over the last decade or so, there have been significant shifts in thinking around child development and behavior and the previously considered more traditional elements of "behavior management." Clinicians and authors such as Dr. Ross Greene, Dr. Dan Siegel, Dr. Bruce Perry, Bo Hejlskov Elvén, Dr. Stuart Shanker, and Dr. Mona Delahooke have used their knowledge of neuroscience and child development to present alternative explanations and approaches for supporting children with behaviors of concern (sometimes referred to as challenging behaviors), approaches that have been particularly relevant for supporting neurodivergent children.

These approaches fit well within the neurodiversity affirming framework, as they acknowledge brain differences and automatic responses of the brain and body in response to stress, and focus on strengths-based supports and environmental accommodations.

One of the biggest shifts in this area is the idea that a child's behavior is adaptive to their situation and the skills they have available to them. Dr. Greene's famous observation, that "kids do well if they can," encourages adults to assume that in any situation, a child is going to do the best they can to solve the problem or get themselves out of danger because children generally want to do the right thing. However, if the most effective skill a child has access to at the time is to hit out or run away, it is likely that they will be seen as acting "inappropriately" when, in fact, they are managing the only way they know how.

When we reframe a child's behavior in this way, we shift away from assuming that a child is in full control of their behavior and acting deliberately to cause problems and move toward a more accepting and developmentally friendly view in which we acknowledge that children are still learning and developing, and need support to build skills to manage challenging situations. In addition to this, it puts the responsibility on the adults involved in a child's care to provide support through co-regulation and accommodations to help a child succeed as they are building the necessary skills.

For example, if a child is frequently involved in conflict with another child in the playground that results in a physical altercation, rather than expecting the child to "manage their emotions better" or "ignore what the other child says," we need to acknowledge that the child currently does not have the skills to manage this situation effectively. Continually putting them back in this situation without support is not going to resolve anything. The child is not suddenly going to learn to do things differently by continuously being placed in a stressful situation. Instead, the adults supporting the child need to put a plan together to support the child in the playground until the child has developed the skills they need, perhaps by facilitating activities, as well as look at ways to assist them to develop the skills necessary to navigate the playground successfully.

Reframing behavior according to neuroscience leads us to a better understanding of how children's brains develop and respond to stress. We all have an inbuilt threat detection system in our brains that is always on the lookout for danger. This is called "neuroception." Neuroception monitors the environment and triggers a stress response in our brains and bodies when danger is detected, a response that is often called "fight, flight, or freeze." This response is automatic and mainly governed by the brainstem and limbic system, involving the release of hormones and physiological changes in the body so that we can be ready to protect ourselves, run away or, in cases where we have no other option, freeze and become unresponsive.

When the brain is in this heightened state, connections between the brainstem and limbic system and the parts of the brain responsible for higher order functions, such as decision-making, problem-solving, reasoning, and learning, are interrupted, making it difficult for a child to "make good choices about their behavior" because the thinking part of their brain is not in control.

In the case of neurodivergence, it appears that neurodivergent children tend to be more reactive to stress due to having brains that are prone to being hypervigilant to threats in their environment. This is likely due to the differences evident in sensory processing, as well as being repeatedly placed in situations in which they are uncertain of what is happening or what is expected of them or being treated poorly by individuals who have not understood their needs. I will discuss this more in the next chapter, in which we will review the intersection of multiple neurodivergences including trauma, but for now, recognizing that neurodivergence tends to involve increased sensitivity to stress is enough.

So how does all this relate to neurodiversity affirming practice? To start with, it recognizes that different brains will respond to situations in different ways depending on their neurotype, developmental level, and abilities. Further, it highlights the need for support and accommodations to assist children to develop the skills they need while also being set up for success rather than putting responsibility on the child to fix things and do better. Third, it emphasizes the fact that a child who is under stress will respond automatically in adaptive ways to a situation, rather than being able to make choices and problem-solve.

This idea that a brain under stress cannot learn is consistent with our earlier discussion of Dr. Perry's model of the 3 Rs (Regulate, Relate, Reason), which suggests that when a child is distressed and does not feel safe or connected to those around them, there is a disconnect between the "survival" part of the brain and higher brain function. This concept certainly makes sense on many different levels, but it is actually life-changing when we consider it from the point of view of traditional behavior management and supporting neurodivergent children with behaviors of concern.

For any of us who have done training in basic behavior management, one of the main premises is that we should not pay attention to or give in to a child who is distressed and seeking attention or wants something, because our behavior will teach the child that if they get upset, they will get what they want. This is based on basic behavioral principles that state that a behavior will increase if it is followed by something pleasurable, and decrease if something negative occurs. To put it simply, a behavior will increase if you reward it and decrease if you punish it.

The problem with this approach is that it was primarily created from studies of animals, and in many cases, it ignores other factors that could influence whether a child engages in a behavior or not, such as their skills, emotions, and environment.

Further, if we consider what modern neuroscience is telling us about how a child's brain operates, if a child is upset, they can't learn in that moment. And if they can't learn in that moment, how will ignoring them or punishing them for becoming distressed stop them reacting that way in the future?

Neurodiversity affirming approaches would suggest that supporting the child in the moment to regulate and process their feelings is the most positive way to manage this situation. It is then our job as adults to problem-solve and determine where the challenges were for the child in this situation, and what we can do to assist them to have success next time. If this means that we need to "give in" and let the child do or have what they want in the moment to help them calm down and prevent an escalation and possible meltdown, then that is okay. This should not be about making a point or having a power struggle; it is about supporting a child and managing a situation as best we can. Then later we can review the situation and plan for next time so we can manage the situation more effectively. Professor Andrew McDonnell, a clinical psychologist with Studio 3 in the UK, has written a fantastic book for therapists that explores the need to be reflective as a clinician and consider new ways of doing things to better support our clients. A link to his book is in the "Useful Resources" section at the end of the book.

In the context of providing therapy, what these new approaches tell us is that we need to focus on regulation and relationships, not rewards and punishments, to support clients in learning to manage their challenges effectively and develop self-confidence and self-worth.

Therapy should not be about forcing a child to comply and do what we tell them just because we are the adult and they are the child. It should be about developing a strong and trusting relationship where a child feels safe and confident in our sessions, and knows that we will work with them to progress and achieve at whatever pace and in whatever way they need.

A NOTE ABOUT REWARDS AND CONSEQUENCES

The use of rewards and consequences has long been considered an essential part of any behavior change program for children. Simply offer the child something they want in exchange for demonstrating a behavior you want to see, or take something away that a child likes if they demonstrate a behavior you don't want, and the child will choose to change their behavior. It really does sound easy, doesn't it?

As I have already mentioned, in reality, there are clearly a lot of factors contributing to a child's behavior, and choice very rarely comes into it. But the whole premise of rewards and punishments hinges on choice—a child must have control of their behavior and be able to make a choice to act a certain way or not, for rewards and punishments to be effective. It is little wonder, then, that research has found that rewards and punishments are largely ineffective.

Reward systems often disadvantage neurodivergent children because they frequently target behaviors that neurodivergent children have difficulty with due to their neurotype, such as sitting in their seat, following instructions, and regulating their emotions.

Even when a child has control over the target behavior (e.g., cleaning their room), and we may see positive changes in the short term when a reward system is put in place, these systems tend not to be effective in the long term. This is because when we rely on extrinsic (external) motivation in the form of a reward, the impact of that reward reduces over time, whereas if we are internally motivated to do something because we enjoy it or it makes us feel good, we are much more likely to continue this in the future.

Another problem with reward systems is that they put the responsibility to change completely on the child, so if the child isn't motivated by the reward or punishment to change their behavior, then it will not work. For example, many parents utilize the threat of "timeout" or sitting on the "naughty step" as a consequence for what they consider bad behavior. The idea is that children won't like being put in timeout and will consequently ensure they behave appropriately at home. While it might sound like a logical system, I have heard many stories of children taking themselves to timeout after they have done something they wanted to do but knew they would get into trouble for. The punishment hasn't stopped the behavior; it just prompted them to think about whether the pay-off for the behavior was worth sitting in timeout for.

It is much better and more effective to form a strong, trusting relationship with a child and to collaborate with them to explore where they are having difficulty. Then we can support them to develop the skills they need to achieve their goals.

Chapter 10

Masking

I think that when most neurotypical individuals think about masking, they mostly think about adapting to situations they are in by tweaking the way they speak and interact, depending on the environment and the social expectations at the time. For example, they might be nervous about a job interview but pretend to be confident and composed to try and make a good impression. Or be completely exhausted but pretend to be excited and switched on when serving a customer at their job. Or perhaps they are required to be quite reserved and serious when in the workplace, but when they are with their friends, they are lively and sociable. This appears to come quite naturally to neurotypical individuals, and could even be considered a common aspect of neurotypical social conventions.

The frequent use of this type of masking in the neurotypical community may be the reason that explains why when the issue of masking comes up with regard to neurodivergent individuals, a common response is "But isn't that a good thing?" or "But we all do that, why is that a problem?" The reason that masking is a problem for neurodivergent individuals is because it is different, and it comes at a high price.

Masking (or camouflaging) in reference to the neurodivergent community describes the act of hiding your authentic self or parts of yourself in an effort to make a particular impression on others or to be accepted socially. This may include suppressing personality traits, neurodivergent characteristics, mental health, or medical symptoms, and temporarily taking on other learned characteristics or behaviors that are seen as more desirable or acceptable in a particular situation.

When neurodivergent individuals mask, it is often because they do not think they will be accepted if they don't. Their experience with the neurotypical community may be such that they have learned that the only way to fit in and be accepted is to pretend to be someone else. For some, this is a constant battle that takes an enormous amount of energy. They may have to think about everything they say and do when in the company of others, holding back impulses or tics, and mimicking facial expressions and body language when they're struggling to follow the conversation, so they don't look out of place. Then afterwards, they often experience a "hangover" when all that effort they had to expend catches up with them, which for some might involve having some screentime to recharge, but for others could involve spending a day or two in bed because of the enormous emotional effort involved in keeping things "together" for so long.

For neurodivergent children, masking may look like the perfect student at school who has a meltdown every night when they get home, or a child who copies the interests, mannerisms, and speech of a classmate or even a popular television character who seems to have lots of friends. Masking can also be more subtle. It could be the child who can't tell their peers they love watching *Thomas the Tank Engine* and pretends they love racing cars instead because their peers will make fun of them. Or the child who bites their nails down to the nail bed because they need to chew something to regulate, and using chewy jewelry will make them look different.

Unfortunately, many neurodivergent children and adolescents are inadvertently encouraged to mask by parents, educators, and clinicians who suggest that a child change the way they interact with their peers so they fit in and are accepted. This is often reinforced further by children being taught neurotypical social skills at school and in group programs. The message these children are really receiving is that they are not worthy of friendship or acceptance the way they are, and that they need to learn to do things the "right" way, which can have a significant negative impact on their self-esteem and self-worth.

For many neurodivergent adults who have masked their whole lives, figuring out how to drop the mask and be themselves is a challenge in itself, because in many cases they have to rediscover who they are when they are not feeling pressured to fit in.

The investment of emotional and physical effort needed to mask has serious consequences for a neurodivergent individual's wellbeing. Further, masking has been shown to lead to negative outcomes for an individual's mental health.

It is essential that clinicians working with neurodivergent children and adolescents are aware of masking and the damage it can do to mental health and wellbeing, so they can support individuals and their families to promote self-acceptance and encourage young people to be their authentic selves in all aspects of their lives.

— Chapter 11 —

Intersectionality

Content Warning: Trauma, suicide.

I believe it is essential in any discussion of neurodiversity and neurodiversity affirming practice that we consider the impact that being multiply neurodivergent, having medical conditions, identifying as being from a minority group, or any combination of these has on an individual's life, and consequently, how we, as therapists, support them.

While it should be considered best practice for clinicians to be aware of a child's medical and developmental history, family, education, and other supports, when a client is neurodivergent there are often many additional factors at play that can interact and intersect in ways that will impact on an individual's ability to engage with therapy, and how they present. In particular, it is important that clinicians do not assume that a concern or challenge identified by a client is solely due to their neurodivergence, and as such is dismissed as not meaningful, when there could be other factors at play.

MENTAL HEALTH

It is well established in research that the incidence of mental health conditions such as anxiety disorders and depression is significantly higher in the neurodivergent community than in the general population. For example, the incidence of clinical levels of anxiety in the Autistic population is around 40 percent compared to around 15 percent in the general population. Further, there are also much higher rates of suicide among neurodivergent individuals including Autistics, ADHDers, Dyslexics, and those with Tourette's syndrome than in the general population, and a higher incidence of substance abuse disorders and addiction.

While it may be assumed by some that mental health concerns are less likely to be a problem for children, this is unfortunately not the case. Due to the challenges neurodivergent children and adolescents face in daily life, they may experience mood fluctuations, anxiety, and poor self-esteem and self-worth, which are already significant concerns; however, many neurodivergent children and teens also experience clinical levels of mental health symptoms that require specific support and treatment.

It is important that clinicians seek out information about how mental health conditions such as anxiety and depression might present in the neurodivergent population, and what the most effective approaches to support them may be. For example, it should not be assumed that individuals with higher support needs, such as those with Intellectual Disability (or Intellectual Developmental Disorder, as it is now referred to in the DSM-5), do not also experience mental health concerns that may need addressing just because their presentation may look different. Thankfully, there are a number of openly neurodivergent clinicians and educators working in this space who are already providing information on this topic for clinicians. A list of resources is included in the "Useful Resources" section at the end of the book.

I can't stress enough the importance of clinicians taking the suicidal ideation of neurodivergent children and adolescents seriously. Again, this may look different to neurotypical children, but it is certainly no less significant. I have had neurodivergent children as young as eight years old tell me that they "don't want to live," that they "don't deserve to be alive," or that everything is so hard they "don't want to do it anymore." Sometimes it is when they are experiencing big emotions or are in the throes of a meltdown that they feel this way; at other times it is an ongoing feeling of despair or desperation for things to change. Even without concrete plans, I have found that the impulsiveness of many neurodivergent children adds additional risk, because even though they may not have a plan to end their life, they may do something in a moment of distress that results in significant harm. It is absolutely vital that these feelings are not just dismissed as something they say but don't mean, but are taken at face value as a cry for help, with a safety plan and supports put in place immediately to assist.

As clinicians, it is essential that we prioritize the mental health of neurodivergent children and adolescents, and recognize that, due to their neurotypes and compounding environmental and societal factors, they are at high risk of developing serious mental health conditions and should be regularly monitored for signs of distress. Addressing the mental health concerns of neurodivergent children and adolescents as they arise will not only support them now, but will also hopefully reduce the likelihood that they will face serious mental health challenges as adults.

TRAUMA

Trauma can be defined as the lasting impact that results from an individual being in a situation in which the emotional and psychological distress experienced is more than the individual's resources (physical, psychological, emotional, relational) can cope with.

For many people, their idea of trauma is a single life-threatening event such as a car accident, fire, or a death. For others, trauma may be associated with ongoing mistreatment and abuse or neglect. However, an event does not have to be what would usually be considered life-threatening to cause trauma. Any exposure to stressful situations in which a child does not have the ability to cope or experiences a persistent lack of control can also be traumatic.

Importantly, we need to remember that it is not the event itself that causes trauma, but the individual's experience and perception of the event, and their ability to access support that will impact whether they are traumatized or not.

It is thought that due to living in a society that is not designed for neurodivergent brains, many neurodivergent children, and in turn, adults, experience trauma from everyday experiences that perhaps other individuals would not find as distressing or on whom they would not have such lasting impacts. Situations such as being bullied by peers at school, repeatedly making social "mistakes" in the playground, being shamed by a teacher for not being able to read or not practicing enough, constantly being reprimanded for impulsive behavior, or having needs and emotions being dismissed and invalidated could result in a child experiencing trauma that in some cases builds and accumulates over time.

When a child experiences repeated adverse events or is exposed to continuous or prolonged negative stress, their brain is exposed to increased levels of stress hormones such as cortisol and adrenaline. This results in the brain being in a heightened state all the time, constantly scanning the environment for threats and being easily triggered into survival mode.

Survival mode (or the Stress response) is an automatic defense mechanism employed by the brain and body to keep us safe. In neurodivergent children, this is often demonstrated as a meltdown or shutdown. A meltdown is often characterized by externalizing behaviors such as screaming, biting, hitting, kicking, throwing things, and running away. In contrast, a shutdown is usually characterized by a child becoming very still, quiet, and unresponsive. In both states the child is highly stressed and is not in control of their actions (see Chapter 15).

One of the most important things to remember when working with neurodivergent children is that it is very likely that they have experienced some trauma and may be reactive to the therapeutic environment or to an adult as therapist. Because a trauma response can be triggered by implicit memories of a situation (e.g., sensory memories rather than conscious recognition of the traumatic experience), children will not always be aware that they are being triggered but may suddenly respond with distress or dysregulation when there is no clear reason. For example, a child who has been repeatedly shamed for their difficulty writing may suddenly go into shutdown when asked to write down some ideas during an activity they were previously engaged in and enjoying. Recognizing these sudden changes in arousal and mood and responding with empathy and curiosity can support a child to regulate in the moment. Building a safe and trusting relationship will further support a child to be able to engage in therapy effectively.

It is important to note that when working with neurodivergent children, it is very likely that we are also working with neurodivergent parents, who may or may not be aware of their neurotype, and may also have a trauma history. This may impact on a parent's ability to participate in their child's therapy and on their engagement with us, as therapists, and we need to ensure that we offer them the same compassion and understanding that we offer their children to help them to also develop a safe and trusting relationship with us.

Taking trauma into consideration when working with neurodivergent children and families is an essential part of providing neurodiversity affirming supports, and will enhance the ability of clinicians to support their clients effectively.

MULTIPLE NEURODIVERGENCE

In my own personal and professional experience, I have found that it is quite common for children and adolescents to be multiply neurodivergent. This may seem like an obvious thing in present times, but it was a relatively short time ago that clinicians were not permitted to identify Autism and ADHD together in an individual, and Intellectual

Disability and Language Disorders were part of the diagnostic criteria for Autism.

Since early 2013, when the *Diagnostic and Statistical Manual of Mental Disorders*, 5th Edition (DSM-5) was released, there have been changes to the way neurodivergence is characterized that have allowed the identification of separate neurotypes and increased awareness of how they interact when present together.

As clinicians, it is important to develop an understanding of the interactions between neurodivergent neurotypes, and I have found the best way to do this is to listen to adults with lived experience, and to speak to our clients about their unique experience of being multiply neurodivergent.

For example, I find that I sometimes experience conflict between my Autistic and ADHD traits where, on the one hand, I have an intense need for organization and predictability, and on the other hand, I have difficulty with the executive functioning required to actually be organized, and struggle to have the ability to stick to a routine. At other times my Autistic and ADHD characteristics seem to complement each other, allowing me to work well under pressure and hyperfocus to get things done. In speaking to other AuDHDer adults (an abbreviation of Autistic and ADHD often used by the neurodivergent community) I have found that many experience the challenges and benefits of their neurodivergent qualities, but they can vary quite considerably between individuals.

Along with combinations of neurodivergences such as Autism and ADHD, and ADHD and Tourette's syndrome, another common combination of neurotypes is Autistic with Verbal Apraxia. Verbal Apraxia is characterized by difficulty with coordinating mouth and speech movements that consequently makes speech challenging and often results in individuals requiring AAC devices to communicate. I wanted to specifically highlight this population of neurodivergent individuals because, in the past, it was often assumed that non-speaking and minimally speaking Autistics were unable to communicate consistently or have independent thought. This is an assumption that has been extremely damaging to many in this community, and has cost many individuals the opportunity to live their lives the way they want due to a lack of understanding and appropriate supports. With the development of better and better AAC devices over the last decade giving non-speaking or minimally speaking Autistics their voices, and the shift in practice to presuming competence, many Autistics with Apraxia are now able to share their experiences and give us an insight into how best to provide them the supports and resources they need to live their best lives.

Being Autistic with Intellectual Disability is another multiply neurodivergent presentation that is prevalent in the neurodivergent community. As you may be aware, Intellectual Disability (or Intellectual Developmental Disorder, as it is now referred to in the DSM-5) can vary in terms of the adaptive behavior challenges an individual faces, from mild to severe, and this can impact significantly on an individual's life. Many individuals with these two neurotypes have high support needs, and require comprehensive and constant daily supports to participate in routine daily tasks such as self-care and personal hygiene, and may present with behaviors of concern such as self-harm and frequent meltdowns. While these individuals may experience considerable challenges and require high levels of care, they are also entitled like anyone else to be given opportunities to learn, pursue interests, participate in recreation activities, and have a good quality of life. It is essential that individuals with high support needs and their families are given the necessary assistance to allow them to achieve success in whatever form that takes.

Obviously, there are many other combinations of neurotypes that can occur in any individual, and for many it is not only one or two but several. Given that many neurodivergent neurotypes are often said to be dynamic, meaning that the intensity and focus of needs change across time and environment, it makes sense that individuals may experience certain neurodivergent traits as being more prominent or challenging at different times, and that some individuals will have significantly higher support needs than others. This is another reason to listen to our clients and their families and be led by them in terms of what they may need the most support with at any one time.

MEDICAL CONDITIONS

There has been increased interest in recent years into medical conditions that appear to have a higher incidence in neurodivergent populations. Research suggests that there are a number of these, although further research continues to be conducted to identify why this might be the case.

Medical conditions that have been identified as more commonly occurring with neurodivergence in adults include Ehlers-Danlos syndrome (EDS) and dysautomnias, such as Postural Orthostatic Tachycardia syndrome (POTS) and Mast Cell Activation syndrome (MCAS).

EDS is actually a group of conditions that affect the connective tissue in the body, with each condition having its own specific characteristics. Common symptoms across all EDS conditions include joint hypermobility, skin hyperextensibility, and tissue fragility, with chronic pain and fatigue.

Dysautomnias are a collection of conditions associated with autonomic nervous system dysfunction that can affect the "automatic" functions of the body such as heart rate, blood pressure, and temperature control. Symptoms of various dysautomnias can include fainting spells, dizziness, unstable blood pressure, sudden fluctuations in heart rate, and fatigue.

MCAS is a condition that involves the repeated triggering of an allergic reaction in the body but without a known cause. Symptoms can be heart-related (e.g., low blood pressure, rapid pulse), skin-related (e.g., itchy rash, hives), lung-related (e.g., shortness of breath, wheezing), and gastrointestinal upset (e.g., diarrhea, nausea).

These conditions can have a significant impact on an individual's daily functioning and quality of life. Given their increased incidence in neurodivergent individuals, it is important that clinicians have an awareness of the symptoms to allow for appropriate referrals to be made when needed.

I think it is relevant when talking about medical conditions to note the difference in pain registration that can be characteristic of some neurodivergent neurotypes, particularly in the Autistic population. While some individuals may experience heightened pain sensations and be able to indicate that they are in pain to receive help, others may experience a very high pain threshold, resulting in a child not registering when they have injured themselves and require support. I have seen this happen with some of my child clients, often with a parent attending the doctors insisting that their child is unwell or hurt but the clinician examining the client not seeing a reaction that would indicate pain or distress. However, on further examination they find that the child has a burst eardrum, or a fractured ankle, and the parent is then blamed for not bringing the child in sooner for treatment, when the child gave little indication there was anything wrong. It is important for any clinicians, but medical practitioners in particular, to be aware of these potential differences in pain registration when examining neurodivergent clients, and ensuring that a reported injury or illness is thoroughly explored.

Further, it is also important to consider signs of pain or illness that may present differently in neurodivergent children who do not have the ability to communicate clearly or who have poor interoception (the ability to understand internal sensations). I often find that a sudden change in a child's behavior, particularly a child who has suddenly become irritable and dysregulated for a day or two with no obvious reason (e.g., no big changes in routine, conflict with peers, etc.), may be becoming unwell and notice something feels different in their body but be unable to pinpoint what it is. Then, when the full symptoms of the illness become evident (e.g., headache, nasal congestion, vomiting, etc.) the reason for the agitation becomes clear. A sudden increase in self-harming behavior can be an indication that a child or adolescent is in pain and needs support. The self-harm may be directed towards the area of pain (e.g., a child repeatedly hitting the side of their head could indicate a headache or earache or tooth pain) or to another area to try and distract or deflect from the pain source.

As clinicians often working with vulnerable clients, it is essential that we pay attention to sudden changes in mood or behavior and listen to the concerns of clients and family members with regard to physical symptoms, to support them to investigate possible medical causes when appropriate, rather than assuming that a symptom or behavior is just part of a child's neurodivergence and not important.

GENDER IDENTITY AND SEXUALITY

The intersection between neurodivergence, gender identity, and sexuality has attracted considerable attention both in the media and in research over the last decade.

For many clinicians who support neurodivergent youth, it probably comes as no surprise that there appears to be a link between neurodivergence and greater sexual diversity. Considerable anecdotal reports by clinicians over the years have pointed to this association, and recent research has confirmed that there is an increased incidence of gender fluidity and differences in sexual orientation in the neurodivergent population, particularly within the Autistic community.

While there are many proposed theories as to why this may be the case, no clear evidence exists that explains the higher rate of neurodivergent individuals that identify as members of the LGBTQI+ community.

Why, then, is this important for clinicians to be aware of?

For neurodivergent children and adolescents, who may still be developing an understanding of their neurodivergence, adding the additional layer of being unsure about their sexual or gender identity can be a source of considerable distress and confusion. Unfortunately, there continues to be stigma and prejudice associated with gender and sexual differences in society, so many young people may be afraid to talk about it or explore what it means for them. Further, being part of intersecting marginalized groups may make our clients more vulnerable to poorer mental health outcomes and increase the risk of suicide.

Having a strong therapeutic relationship and being neurodiversity affirming in our approach makes it more likely that a young person may feel safe to open up to a clinician and share their feelings or ask questions they haven't been able to ask anywhere else. This provides us with an opportunity to acknowledge and validate our clients' feelings, reassure them that it is okay to be unsure or have different feelings about sexuality and gender, and support them to obtain reliable and appropriate information.

Providing support around sexuality and gender may not be something that fits within your clinical role, and that is okay. However, it is important to understand these issues, and to think about how you would respond to a young person who shares their feelings with you. Being open, curious, and empathetic to your client sharing such personal and important information will likely make it easier for them to speak to others about it and seek support in the future.

For clinicians who are unable to support a client on their journey in the longer term, referring a client on to affirming services that support the LGBTQI+ community and that understand neurodivergence will be important.

I think it is necessary to add here that not all neurodivergent youth who are unsure about their sexuality and gender will require specialized supports. For a client who identifies as transgender, attending a specialist gender clinic to assist with various needs such as possible medication, gender dysphoria, and plans for transition would be important. However, for a client who is exploring their gender identity or sexuality and is comfortable with who they are, they may just need time and the support of family and friends to figure out their preferences and feel confident to be themselves.

ETHNICITY AND CULTURE

I would like to conclude this chapter about intersectionality by discussing an extremely important topic: ethnicity and culture.

Neurodivergence does not discriminate between ethnicity or culture, and nor does it discriminate between socioeconomic status or education. Neurodivergence is part of the human condition, and as a natural variation in neurotype, it can be seen everywhere. However, where a child is born and who they are born to may impact on whether their neurodivergence is identified, whether appropriate assessments and supports are available, and how their neurodivergence is perceived by their community.

I am fully aware that as a white woman who has a supportive family, a world-class education, and is financially stable, I am in a position of privilege. When seeking identification and support for my youngest son many years ago, I was able to readily access professionals who could guide me in understanding him and providing what he needed so he could thrive. In my own life, I have been able to pursue my passions, receive support when I have needed it, and have been able to seek out and obtain a professional assessment to identify my neurotypes when I was ready. Unfortunately, for many individuals seeking identification and support for themselves or their family members in other parts of society or other parts of the world, all of this might seem, or actually be, impossible.

Where I live in Australia, the neurodiversity affirming movement is gaining attention and followers, gradually bringing with it a better understanding and acceptance of neurodivergence. However, in some other parts of the world, neurodivergence is firmly rooted in the medical model and is seen as a mental disorder, often with significant stigma attached. This may result in families avoiding assessment and identification of neurodivergence in an effort to protect their child and family from shame in their community.

Even in places where neurodiversity is being embraced, there are inherent challenges in making assessment and identification of neurodivergence accessible to anyone who needs it. Diagnostic services are full and running waitlists, families are sometimes waiting years to get access to a clinician for assessment, and there are many families who would not be able to afford the assessment process even if they could get in to see someone.

On top of problems with access to assessment, the reality is that most diagnostic tools, like many other psychological assessments, have been based on Western norms, and as such do not have the sensitivity to distinguish differing presentations across cultures. This may result in the over- or under-identification of neurodivergence of children in different ethnic groups and in different parts of the world.

It is essential that clinicians working with diverse populations develop cultural competence, and consider the beliefs and possible stigma associated with neurodivergence in some cultures when supporting children and families. For example, a family may be open to their child being identified as Autistic but be unable to disclose their child's neurodivergence and care needs to extended family due to the stigma involved, and may consequently have no family support they can rely on. We can develop our cultural competence by listening to our clients' experiences as well as seeking out information and guidance from cultural elders and other community leaders to ensure we are providing the most culturally sensitive supports to our clients and families.

It is important to consider individual needs within the context of a child and family's culture when suggesting and providing therapies. While in a perfect world we would be able to ensure that all children could fully be their neurodivergent selves without fear of stigma or mistreatment, there may be situations in which a child may need to learn to mask or comply with authority without question to ensure their safety. For example, many ethnic minorities in predominantly white communities may be in danger of harm if they exhibit openly autistic behaviors and do not follow the direction of law enforcement immediately. In a case like this, it would still be important to work with the child and family in an affirming way, but possibly build these skills into the child's repertoire as a protective element.

While the topics listed in this chapter were not exhaustive, I hope they have given you an idea of the possible complexities of working with neurodivergent clients. I believe it is essential that we do not see neurodivergence in isolation, and instead consider other factors in a child or adolescent's life that may have an impact on their needs and how we provide support.

Chapter 12

Supporting and Educating Parents

Just as the idea of neurodiversity affirming practice is new to many professionals, it is also a new concept for many parents and families.

The identification of a child as neurodivergent is often associated with negative connotations, I think in part due to the fact that parents are usually seeking a diagnosis for their child at a time when the child and family are experiencing significant challenges, or have concerns that a child does not fit the norm with regard to communication, social interaction, play, learning, or behavior. Consequently, the focus from the very beginning of a child and family's journey becomes the child's deficits and challenges, and this continues throughout childhood and adolescence as the fight for services, supports, and funding invariably requires further deficit-focused discussion. Unfortunately, this negative view is often also reinforced by professionals who are still entrenched in the medical model of disability.

I am slowly seeing this attitude change as parents become more aware of neurodivergence, and are seeking identification for help in understanding how best to support their child and to help their child understand themselves, but this is still a relatively rare occurrence.

As I have said several times already throughout this book, being neurodiversity affirming does not mean seeing neurodivergence through rose-colored glasses and only seeing the positives or ignoring distress or discomfort; it is about honoring and respecting the individual's neurotype and the qualities that are inherent in their neurodivergence, and supporting them with any challenges they face to make life better and easier. It is about everyone having the same opportunities and access to services and supports, and the right to be safe, connected, and valued in the community.

I have heard it said by some parents of children and adolescents with very high support needs that the neurodiversity affirming movement doesn't represent them, that it is only individuals who can advocate for themselves and who are able to be independent that benefit from this narrative. I don't see it that way. I see being neurodiversity affirming as a way to provide opportunities to everyone, including those with significant needs, to live their best lives with whatever support they require to achieve this.

So, when we are talking about being neurodiversity affirming with families and supporting them to seek out affirming supports and resources, it is important that we acknowledge and seek to understand their challenges as well as promote an affirming outlook and approach to accepting their child's differences and addressing their needs.

Our role in supporting parents to understand neurodiversity affirming practice starts in their very first interaction with us, regardless of whether they already know their child is neurodivergent or they are coming to see us to explore that possibility. The way parents hear us talk about neurodivergence will make a difference to their outlook and, in turn, the way their child sees their differences, so it is essential that we frame their child's neurotype in a positive and affirming way.

To begin with, we want to support parents to understand that neurodivergence represents a natural variation in neurotypes or brain types, and that all different types of brains are beneficial to society and have strengths and challenges. This can be a good time to discuss the different qualities of neurodivergent brains, and how being able to think differently and perceive the world differently is necessary for society to progress. For example, neurodivergent brains have always been with us throughout history. Neurodivergent individuals may be very creative, have strengths in visual processing and attention to detail, be amazing problem-solvers, have strengths in drama and debating, be very caring and empathic, and may have a wicked sense of humor. Unfortunately, many parents I work with have become so used to identifying their child's challenges that they can struggle to describe their child's strengths. We need to help parents to see the positive qualities their child has, but this is not always easy.

For parents who are seeing their child struggling with different aspects of life such as with emotional regulation, learning, self-care, or social interaction, it may still be hard to see the positives. No parent wants to see their child struggle. Parents want what is best for their children, and when things seem to be going wrong and their child is having difficulties, they worry for their child's future. Even more than that, if parents have experienced challenges themselves in their childhood, they may feel even more distressed about the possibility that their child is going to have to go through what they went through, and it might be hard to shift their thinking to be hopeful. I find the best way to support parents with developing an affirming outlook is to help them see their child's individual strengths, acknowledge the challenges they may face, and reassure them that we now know so much more about how to support neurodivergent children and adults, that they will hopefully not face the same barriers that children faced in the past, and will have the opportunity to be who they want to be.

It can also be helpful for parents to understand the social model of disability and the idea of neurodivergence as a cultural difference. This can help frame the idea that whatever their child's strengths and challenges, with the right supports and opportunities, neurodivergent individuals can find their place in the world and thrive.

Some parents may push back with the idea that the world isn't just going to change for their child and that their child is going to have to face the harsh realities of a world that isn't built for them.

They may even insist that making accommodations for them now will not prepare them adequately for adulthood, and so they just need to learn how to cope. It is important if this occurs that we acknowledge a parent's concerns and bring things back to facts about the child's abilities and development. We need to support parents to understand that their child will continue to learn and develop but will also likely require some supports into adulthood, and that setting them up now for success with the right assistance will prepare them for later on. It can be helpful during these discussions to highlight the kinds of accommodations and supports that we, as adults, often put in place for ourselves to assist us to manage our daily lives, and to recognize that children are generally not offered that level of autonomy, and so we need to put accommodations in place for them. For example, in the workplace we might get up and stretch and make a cup of coffee whenever we feel the need to move, whereas at school children are generally expected to sit in their seat for long periods and must ask permission to move or get a snack. Further, as adults we can use spell check, predictive text, and recently even artificial intelligence (AI) to help us write letters and documents, and use "text-to-speech" to have our computers read to us, whereas at school we are expected to do all of these things without assistance, and are penalized when we don't produce work to the quality that is expected. We need to normalize the need for accommodations and remove the ableist shame associated with needing support.

Another important element to supporting parents is to help them understand that identifying neurodivergence and supporting their child to understand how their brain works is helpful and leads to better outcomes in young people. At times parents are worried about children receiving labels, and that this may put them at some sort of disadvantage or carry stigma. The reality is that children who do not know about their neurodivergence until later in life overwhelmingly tell us that they thought there was something wrong with them, and that identification helped them understand and accept who they were. Further, with identification also comes the possibility of finding other children and adults like them, and developing a sense of belonging, which can be a protective factor against future mental health concerns.

Finally, it is important to encourage parents to seek out lived experience experts to help them gain an insight and understanding of real neurodivergent experiences. Just as clinicians can learn from the neurodivergent community, parents can also benefit immensely from hearing the stories of neurodivergent individuals to provide insight and different perspectives that can help them better understand the experiences of their children.

— Chapter 13 —

Self-Advocacy

One part of neurodiversity affirming practice that may not necessarily seem like a clinician's role, but I think is extremely important, is to support clients to develop self-advocacy skills.

Clinicians might be used to advocating for clients to receive accommodations at school or home, or to support them to access external funding or assistance, but self-advocacy is an important skill that we can support our clients to develop.

The opportunity for a client to self-advocate is built into neurodiversity affirming practice. If we presume competence, promote autonomy, and respect all communication styles, then clients will be given the opportunity at every stage to advocate for themselves with their clinicians. In providing clients with these opportunities and being receptive and respectful of their decisions, we are showing them that their voice matters and that their wants and needs are important. However, we also want our clients to have the tools and the confidence to advocate for themselves and their needs in other settings, and this can be particularly difficult for children and adolescents to do.

In its simplest form, self-advocacy starts with being able to communicate "yes" or "no" in words or actions or with AAC. If an individual can communicate whether or not they want to do something, are interested in something, or like something, this can be used as a tool to self-advocate. "No" can be an incredibly powerful word, even for very young children. But to learn to communicate this, and understand that they can have a say in what happens to them, a child or adolescent has to be given choices and have their preference acknowledged. Unfortunately, this is not always something that is offered, especially to children. Further, there is often a power imbalance between a child or adolescent and any adult involved in their care, which means that opportunities to self-advocate may only be possible if the adult makes them available. While we can't force other adults to offer the same opportunities to our clients as we do, we can educate them by modeling and discussing neurodiversity affirming practice, and making it clear that our client is involved in decision-making about their care. In this way we can promote our clients' ability to self-advocate with others.

For children and adolescents who can communicate their needs more specifically (e.g., phrase speech, writing in phrases or sentences, AAC), it is important to first help them to understand their strengths and challenges, and to then identify what they need in order to participate in activities and to accommodate their challenges effectively. Clinicians can do this by exploring what the child does well and what they might need help with at home, at school, and in the community. Then clinicians can work with them to reflect on what has helped them in the past or what they wish was available to them to make life easier. This may be difficult for some children to discuss and reflect on, but I find that children often have much more insight than we give them credit for. Clinicians need to be open to exploring their experiences with clients and being curious about what works best in their world. Some children may not be able to tell you what works, but they will be very clear on what doesn't work for them, or what they find difficult, which is very useful information. For those children who really are not sure what is helpful for them, or where they might need support, it is good to work with them using a bit of trial and error to figure out what supports resonate with them or not. In that way we can help clients build up a toolbox of accommodations and supports that they are confident are helpful to them. Working through this process with clients will also give them experience with a problem-solving model that they can use to identify possible new supports in the future as their needs change.

Once a child has a sense of what helps them in different situations, or even just recognizes that they need help, clinicians can guide the child in how to communicate this to others when they need support. For example, clinicians can work with the child to develop and practice short scripts or examples of what they can say to advocate for themselves. This may be asking for help, saying they need a break, or telling an adult how they learn best (e.g., "I need to sit on a chair at mat time" or "Using my fidgets helps me listen"). For children who use AAC or are minimally verbal, sometimes the use of pictures or cards that communicate needs and can be shown to a teacher or another adult can be useful (e.g., a card that has "I need a break" printed on it).

Clinicians can also support clients to build their confidence to advocate for themselves by giving them a voice in meetings and planning with teachers and other caring adults. This might be through collaborating with clients to include their perspective or opinion in reports and letters to educators or professionals. It could be through encouraging clients to write a letter or record a video to introduce themselves to a new teacher and explain how they learn best and what they need in the classroom. It might even be through facilitating a meeting between a client and their teacher or principal to discuss how a school can best support the client's needs. In whatever way they feel comfortable, clinicians can support clients to have their voices heard.

Supporting clients to self-advocate helps clinicians to act in accordance with what clients want and need rather than just recommending what we think is best. It also helps others see that our clients have a right to be listened to and have consideration given to what they say. For example, I recently worked with several of my clients to create transition letters to support them moving into secondary school. I began each letter stating that my client had given me permission to provide information (e.g., "I am writing with Sally's permission to provide you with some additional information about her support needs..."), and also stated that I had collaborated with my client on what supports were needed (e.g., "The following list of supports has been created in collaboration with Sally..."). In this way I could acknowledge the input that was given by my clients, and show the school that my clients were involved in the process and should be included in discussions about their supports.

I should note here that even when children and adolescents are successful in advocating for themselves, there needs to be a willing communication partner who is responsive to them for their efforts to be effective. Unfortunately, this is not always going to be the case. Clinicians can prepare clients for the possibility that they will occasionally be faced with adults and peers who will not listen or be responsive to their needs, and we can help them to seek further support from a trusted adult in these situations to assist them to have their needs met. Clinicians can also ensure that the adults involved in a child's care are aware that the child is being encouraged to self-advocate where possible, and how they can respond to support the child in an affirming way.

— PART 3 —

IN PRACTICE

In this section I would like to provide you with an overview of how to approach therapy from a neurodiversity affirming standpoint. Please note that this section isn't designed to provide specific therapy activities, but is more about providing a general understanding of how a neurodiversity affirming approach may make us look at particular aspects of therapy from a different direction, and to guide you to be able to identify whether something you are working on would be considered neurodiversity affirming or not.

— Chapter 14 —

What Do Neurodivergent Children Want from Therapy?

I have been privileged throughout my career so far to work with many amazing neurodivergent young people who have allowed me to be part of their lives to offer them support and guidance, and who have shared their experiences and taught me along the way as well. Every young person I work with teaches me something through our journey together that I carry with me to make me a better clinician, and I value those lessons immensely.

It was important to me that I did not just share what I have learned about neurodiversity affirming practice with you all, but that I also shared the voices of the young people I work with to help you understand things from their point of view about what being a neurodiversity affirming therapist looks like.

To help me do this, I invited Chloe M, a 13-year-old Autistic ADHDer, to share her experiences of therapy and ideas for making therapy more neurodiversity affirming. Chloe is an aspiring advocate for children with disabilities, and is already using her experiences to help others and instigate change. I feel that it is important to note here that Chloe and her mother both gave informed consent to participate in an interview for this book, and Chloe was compensated for her contribution.

So first, let me introduce you to Chloe.

Chloe is an intelligent, insightful and creative 13-year-old Autistic ADHDer. She is a huge fan of all things Pokémon, and also loves animals, science, and art. She lives in Australia with her mother, father, and younger sister, all of whom are neurodivergent, and her three dogs. Chloe also has medical diagnoses of Postural Orthostatic Tachycardia syndrome, Inappropriate Sinus Tachycardia, Generalized Anxiety Disorder, and Specific Phobia. She has a long history of frequent medical appointments and procedures, as well as regular psychology, speech pathology, and physiotherapy.

I interviewed Chloe over two one-hour sessions. While Chloe's experiences and opinions are her own, they reflect the experiences and needs of countless children and adolescents I have worked with over many years, and who regularly express similar concerns.

For ease of reading and flow, I have edited some aspects of my conversation with Chloe for clarification and put in subheadings to highlight themes; however, the quotes from Chloe are hers alone.

THERAPY

To start our interview, I asked Chloe about her experiences with therapy and what qualities she looks for in a therapist:

> Someone who can make it into more of a conversation than therapy. That's what I like. It's more like you can get your thoughts and stuff out by having a conversation rather than other ways [of doing therapy].

We reflected on Chloe's early therapy experiences, particularly in psychology, which often involved learning about specific things such as thoughts and feelings, and I asked Chloe if she felt like that was helpful:

Well, when I was younger and really only just starting to learn it. Yes. But once I had learned a lot about it, I came to prefer the conversations. Conversations of what's happened during the week and ways we can work around that.

Chloe went on to clarify that she liked being able to talk about situations and problem-solve and have more of a relationship with her therapist where they could just have a conversation rather than it being like a teacher and student, where the interaction might be more questions and answers. She said she liked the idea of just being able to relate and chat while she was doing what she needed to do. Whether that was exercising or practicing something or doing something, it was helpful to be able to do it while chatting:

> Yeah. For example, I might like to have a conversation about how I've been struggling over the week and discuss that and discuss ways that I could maybe work on things, strategies to help. But I'd also like to have conversations sometimes about what's going on with Pokémon.

I asked Chloe whether she likes to just sit and talk, or whether she prefers to be doing something while she chats:

> I like to be doing something while I'm doing it too. I could focus... For example, I might do coloring to help me focus compared to just sitting here. 'Cause otherwise I'm not going to be able to focus.

Chloe mentioned that with her speech pathologist she plays Nintendo Switch, and with her physical therapist she focuses on movement. There is always something happening in addition to talking:

> To help it just naturally flow... So, it's almost a bit of side by side talking rather than sitting opposite each other, having to look at

each other and talk because it just really feels relaxed. Like I can come here and just talk.

Given that Chloe emphasized the importance of doing something while talking, and the pressure there might be to make eye contact while talking in some environments, I asked Chloe if eye contact was important to her:

No. It never has been. Never will be. Yeah.

Then Chloe mentioned a recent interaction with her physical therapist who she loves, and who really understands her and her needs. She explained that her therapist had checked in with her about her understanding of her nervous system and how anxiety works, and when Chloe indicated she understood, the therapist moved on to doing some movement and exercise.

I asked Chloe whether she felt it was important for therapists to recognize what knowledge and experience clients bring to therapy:

Yes, if that person already has a great toolbox, then they don't need to go over that all over again. And instead, just going onto doing, for example, with [the therapist] doing the physical therapy and just having fun with it. She'd still talk about some of it, but it was always while we were doing it and very much in a conversational way of, "This is helping, this..."

Chloe went on to explain the importance of clinicians focusing on a client's individual needs:

And another thing is having someone who focuses on the individual compared to everyone else they're working with. And focusing on that individual person and that individual person's needs compared to looking at another person they're working with and doing exactly the same thing for the other person that they were doing with that one... I think it's great to focus, it's great to take stuff that you've done with someone else and give advice as how you've done this with someone else, then it might work for you. But if it doesn't that's fine. And you find something else that might work. Because it's different for everyone.

I clarified with Chloe that she was happy for clinicians to mention trying something that they had seen work with another client to see if it might work for them, but not to give the client one option and say they need to do it that way without recognizing that they might need something different:

It's much better to just focus on "this may work for you, but if not, let's try something else." Because there isn't just one option. There are so many different ways to help.

Next, we went back to discussing Chloe's early therapy experiences. I asked Chloe if she felt that the way we learned about concepts and practiced skills was helpful then:

When I was younger, I remember we used to read a whole lot of books and go over stuff from inside the books. So, for example, if it was a topic of anxiety and the book had things about how anxiety might affect you, we would focus on what was inside that book. But now I know so much about anxiety that I don't really need to do that anymore.

I asked Chloe about the structure of her sessions with other therapists, and if having structure was helpful to make sessions predictable:

Yeah. But everyone was also a little bit different in how they did it... It was just a different style. And it was still working for me because it was how I needed things. But just a little bit different because it's the individual person. That's just how it works.

THERAPEUTIC RELATIONSHIPS

Chloe and I have had discussions on many occasions about the importance of having strong trusting relationships with the clinicians she sees. I asked her what she thought was the best way for a therapist to build a strong relationship with a client:

> It may be doing some of that therapy and then having a discussion about one of their favorite things. For example, with me, I like to do therapy and then I might have a discussion at the end about what the latest Pokémon news is. And just have that conversation and it's not really therapy. It's more like bonding.

I was interested to know what other ways Chloe felt that therapists could develop trust in their relationships with clients:

> Well, another way is being able to have someone who I can come to and just express how I've been feeling throughout the week and just say how good the week's been or how bad the big week's been. And just get that out and not feel like there's some judgment there. I'm allowed to just get it out. Yeah. And not be judged with it.

Chloe went on to explain how a therapist could let clients know that they were not being judged, and that it was safe for them to talk about their experiences:

> If they sometimes respond with relatable comments on how they might have had similar events throughout the week or had stuff happen that has affected them as well and not just, not just being about the, what would you call it? Like client?

Chloe also talked about the importance of therapists acknowledging and validating a client's experience so they know that they are really being heard, rather than needing the therapist to immediately try and fix the problem, or having them justify the actions of others that might have caused distress:

> Just more of a back and forth conversation of "Yeah, that's really bad. It's like a really bad week you've had, or a great week you've had." Like, whatever it is, it is just responding with that. For example, if it was a bad week "Yeah. You've just had a really bad week, it's okay. Like everyone has bad weeks." And it's not dismissing it. It's acknowledging without trying to immediately fix and maybe defend. Yeah. Defend why and defend the others. And just acknowledging that "It's just been a bad week, hasn't it?"

In our previous discussions, Chloe had mentioned that having a therapist sharing a little bit of themselves was important to maintaining or establishing a connection. I asked her how she felt about this:

> It doesn't have to happen, but it is something that can definitely really help build that relationship because you feel like it's not just about you. And instead, it's like they're sharing things that happened with them and, you know, just having that connection.

Even when clients feel connected, it can take a while for them to get comfortable and be able to unmask and be their true selves with clinicians. I asked Chloe how long she thinks it could take for neurodivergent clients to unmask:

> It definitely doesn't happen immediately. It can take some time. But like, now I've probably only just started to really unmask. Well not just now, but it's probably only been within the past two years that I've only just started to really unmask and just get confident in talking to you and (my speech pathologist). It's a very slow process, but once you get there it's worth it because

you just feel like you can just unmask and just feel great and not have to...

Chloe then shared her thoughts on why it is important for clinicians to persist with clients who seem difficult to get to know or who won't initially open up:

Because that's just what neurodivergent people do, they mask... And often sometimes they don't even know they're masking. It just happens and they only start to unmask once they gain their trust. And once they actually believe that whoever it is going to be able to let them unmask and not judge them. And the best thing that I think a therapist can do is not just stop trying to build that relationship because whoever it is isn't giving you anything. You keep going because they're going to give you something one day. And that's going to be what starts to build that relationship.

They're not going to say stuff immediately. You need to let them say stuff eventually. And let that relationship build before you just say no because...you don't just give up because they're not giving you anything. You keep going and you keep showing them that you are there to have that space and give them that time. So that they feel okay to unmask and build that relationship. Because if you don't, if you stop giving them that, they're not going to ever unmask and they're going to always stay masked up because...you stop giving them that trust.

SETTING GOALS

Next, I wanted to talk about goal-setting and get Chloe's perspective on how goals are created and worked on in therapy. Chloe had also told me in the past that she doesn't like the idea of goals, so I wanted to understand why this was a difficult subject for her. I asked her what it is about goals that she doesn't like:

> You know what? Some kids probably don't want goals. And you know what? I personally don't want any goals. My goal is just to get through the day.
>
> I don't like goals. I don't like having a goal for writing and a goal for school because my goal is to just function for the year and get through a day. So, sometimes I'll have something I want to work towards in the future and I will decide I want to do this. But I may get it done, I may not.

I wondered whether the issue was that goals often have a time limit and the expectation of completion within that time, and if a goal being meaningful to her was important:

> Yeah, because goals are very much, you set a time frame for it, whereas, you know just achieving something, I want to just achieve this now. And I'm not going to work towards something that I don't want to work towards. Because then am I going to get it done? Nope.

After establishing that Chloe preferred the idea of "tasks" or a "focus for sessions" instead of using the word "goals," I asked Chloe what she thought would be the best way to decide on a focus for sessions so that the therapist and the client can work together:

> If the therapist comes in with an idea and the person doesn't want to do that and has a different idea, they will have to respect that and do whatever the client wants. And you know what, sometimes the client may not have an idea. They may be happy to do whatever the therapist wants. It may be just if there's an

idea there, they can work it out together, work out what they'd like to do for the day.

I was interested in what Chloe thought therapists should do when a parent's focus for sessions was different to what clients wanted to do:

> Don't force the kid into it, but sometimes it may be worth trying to convince them. Because I know for [my sister], she will come in and she will not want to do therapy, but there will be something that we really want to work on, and she may not want to do it so we don't force it.

Chloe reflected that if the parent's idea of something to work on would benefit the client, it might be worth talking to the client about how it would be useful to do that. She suggested working on what the client wanted to focus on, but introducing other elements when appropriate:

> And if the client is very stuck, sometimes it can be helpful just discreetly getting that conversation in there somehow. Put it into a discussion. One thing I know is that sometimes I can get very stuck on, "but I want to do this." And sometimes I will end up talking about the other thing just because we were having a conversation about something and somehow that was brought into it. And that feels fine. It's like I was able to talk about what I wanted, and I was also able to talk about something that needed to be talked about.

AUTONOMY

I wanted to hear from Chloe about her experience with doctors and specialists who she may not have the opportunity to form strong relationships with. I asked Chloe what clinicians can do to make clients more comfortable in their appointments. I also reminded her that she had previously mentioned having clinicians explaining what they are doing as being helpful:

> Yes... For example, if they're going to do a needle and something, you don't just do the needle. You say to them that, "Okay, we're going to do the needle," and tell them where you are and where you are touching so that they don't get a fright. So then the people don't get a fright and panic because they've all of a sudden been touched or jabbed with the needle. But at the same time, some people like countdowns, others don't. You always ask what they need and don't just assume. If they say that they would prefer not to see the needle, you don't show them the needle. If they say that they don't want a countdown, you don't give them a countdown. If they said that they do, you give them a countdown. You ask what they need, and you work with that because they know what they need.

Chloe put a lot of emphasis on the clinician asking clients what they need and being receptive to what they are being told:

> Asking, yes. You ask what it is they need. Because you can't just assume that they might need this or that and just do it. And then that panics them, and they get a bad experience out of that and never want to come back again. And they may actually get a phobia because of that experience or start to become afraid of going to the doctors because of one experience that they've had where they weren't asked if they were okay with it. It's always about what the person says they need. And even with kids, they can know what they need too, and the parents, too, will know what the kids need, and you listen to that. You listen to what they say they need.

HONESTY

Chloe also explained the importance of being told the truth by therapists:

> That is just a general thing of life and conversation. Doctors should always say the truth...if you say that you're not going to do the needle and you all of a sudden do the needle, then that's going to really panic them and that's going to cause some trust issues. Whereas if you were to just say that you're going to do the needle and do whatever they need for that needle, then all issues are gone. You've done what they need. And in therapy, if you were to lie about something working, but it doesn't work then... You give exactly the information that is happening. And if there's been an issue with something along the lines, you say to them, there's been an issue, we need to work this out. We'll take accountability. If you've done something wrong, that's okay. You just need to admit you've done something wrong, and everything will be fine because it's when you don't admit it that there's problems.

I asked Chloe why it was important for therapists to acknowledge when they had made a mistake or got something wrong:

> Often all I need is an apology and then it's all okay because I've gotten the apology. They've acknowledged they've done something wrong and have said that they never meant to, and that they will try not to again. Because then I don't start to think that they've done it on purpose. If a situation like that happens, I might actually think that they've done it on purpose, and it hasn't just been an accident because I haven't gotten an apology for it. If I don't get that then I'm not going to know and I'm automatically going to start thinking the worst.

EATING IN THERAPY

During her interview, Chloe made a point of bringing up something that has come up in appointments and has caused a lot of frustration—the topic of eating during therapy:

> Another thing I want to mention...eating food in therapy is not at all disrespectful. The only time it's disrespectful is if the person's allergic to the food you're eating.

I asked Chloe whether she found eating helpful because it's regulating or because if she is hungry, she needs to eat and that's going to make her feel better:

> Both. And waiting until the end of the session is not going to be helpful because you're going to get anxious, stressed, hungry.

BEING INVOLVED IN APPOINTMENTS

Next, I wanted to talk to Chloe about attending appointments and how involved she is able to be. I asked her if she had ever been in a situation where she had been ignored and the therapist has just talked to Mum or Dad and pretended she wasn't there:

> Regularly! The doctors I like are the ones who say "Hi" to me because I'm the patient. And they're working with me and they're working on my stuff, so I'd like to be said hello to. And I'd like to be given an introduction... I mean, I feel like you want that from anyone. If I'm too nervous to talk, then let Mum and Dad talk because I don't have the words and Mum and Dad do. And often I don't exactly know why I'm there. I'm kind of just there because I need to be.

I wondered whether Chloe would prefer that a clinician checked with her if they saw she couldn't talk. Perhaps to ask her if it's okay if Mum and Dad let them know what is going on or do the talking:

> Yeah. So that I'm not pressured to be having to answer anything... it calms my nerves. So I don't have to worry too much about answering questions. I know that if I can't do that, Mum and Dad can. So that I'm allowed to be part of a conversation if I want to, but not pressured to be.

I asked Chloe what she thought of situations where a clinician talks to a parent in front of her without her being acknowledged:

> Well, I'm still in the room. I'm still there, so if you're going to talk about me, at least allow me to join into the conversation if I want to because I'm there. You are talking about me and if something's been said wrong and I want to correct that, then I would like to be able to.

> I think it's okay to talk about them in front of them if they're aware of the things that you're talking about. If you're going to talk about them in front of them and they have no idea what's happening or like they might overhear things and get worried, that's not right.

Then I asked Chloe about the impact of a parent and clinician talking about problems with what a child is doing in front of the child:

> You don't want the child to be there because they're not going to be okay with that happening. There's a fine line of stuff you'd say in front of the child and don't say in front of the child. And if you're going to say stuff in front of the child that they may not want to hear or something, depending on what it is, you either

avoid saying that until next time or send an email. The child understands a lot more than you think.

I commented to Chloe that even when a child doesn't understand the words that are being used, they do understand if there is tension and the tone of voice of the people in the room. Chloe added that they would also understand the body language:

They know that whatever's being talked about them isn't a great thing.

THE IMPORTANCE OF LISTENING AND COLLABORATING

I wanted to find out from Chloe specifically about her journey investigating her health conditions. I asked her what she has found most helpful in terms of her interactions with medical specialists:

One of the biggest things is finding a specialist that listens. Goodness, it is hard sometimes.

An example is pain. My pain specialist was very, very dismissive. "Oh, but you have Autism, you have all the sensory stuff, that would be enhancing all your pain." I can tell you the difference between my pain, my POTS pain, and my anxiety pain very directly. If you listen to me, you'd know that this is not anxiety, this is not enhanced. This is like I'm living every day with excruciating pain. So, it's very much do not dismiss it because I'm not *not* in pain. I'm in extreme pain. I'm very much experiencing the symptoms of POTS. But them getting very dismissive about it is not great.

Having a specialist who listened and didn't dismiss Chloe's concerns was clearly a big factor in her satisfaction with medical specialists. I asked her what else she felt was important in making her experience a positive one. Chloe talked about making testing as easy as possible by combining pathology visits and tests, and also being mindful of a client's sensitivities when talking about particular topics:

> Being very understanding of the fact that if you need to get...if someone has a fear of needles, if you need to get blood tests done, do as many as you can at once. Rather than have several needles throughout the entire month that you're kind of, like, why can't we just do this all in the same day? And people who are very much not great with hearing things about the body and things. If that person says that they can't actually hear any more, listen to them. Because I know for one, when I have to do things like going to the heart specialist, they talk a lot about blood stuff and hearing that, sometimes it gets far too much and I can't hear anymore. If I say that I need you to stop...and sometimes it can also be, if you're talking about something, sometimes you need to be very careful with the language you use. If that person has a phobia of blood, for example, be careful with how much you use the word.

Chloe also wanted to comment on the differences between clinicians' willingness to provide a diagnosis and the need for sharing information with patients and collaborating:

> And one thing that I've found is sometimes the doctors will be, like, will be, so the geneticist we're currently seeing is very cautious about diagnosing us with anything. And I appreciate that and it's great that he is, but personally I'm kind of, like, can I just get the diagnosis, I have the thing. But for some people they may want that. So do that for them. But don't just give them the diagnosis. Kind of ask if they really feel like that's what they have. If they, like, for example, have POTS, do you really feel like you

have POTS? Do you feel that that's what you have and ask them? Because once you put that on paper, that's not coming out easily.

And it can also be helpful to be really informative and inform them of things that could happen with that. Not particularly for the diagnosis side of it, but once you get the diagnosis of, again, POTS, it's a good example of saying that here are some of the things you can experience with it. Here are some of the things we can give you to help with that. And just kind of going, we can help with this. And giving advice and that kind of stuff. I'm going to be really honest, the doctor's stuff, Mum deals with a whole lot more than I do. I kind of just go to the appointment, I sit there, I watch my iPad and go, I have this diagnosis. Cool. What meds am I on now?

I reflected that Chloe not always being involved in the appointment was completely okay as the important thing was her having a choice. If she chooses not to be involved, that is what she needs to do in that moment:

Just gimme the choice. If I want to be involved, I'll get involved. If not, yeah. I'll sit there quietly watching my iPad. Because sometimes I don't really want to get involved. And I don't really want to deal with it because, you know, sometimes it's not easy to hear about it. And also, kind of, I don't really want to be listening to all this professional doctor's stuff about exactly what results my blood test got. I'll just sit on my iPad. I am a child; I don't need to know about any test.

INTERSECTIONALITY

Given that Chloe is multiply neurodivergent and experiences a number of health conditions, I thought it was important to talk to her about the idea of intersectionality, and whether she felt that the clinicians involved in her care had an understanding of how her neurotypes and health might impact each other:

> I find that there often isn't a really good understanding between all of it. Mostly because most of them have their own special area and they don't really know about this other area. And it's kind of like they just assume. Stop assuming. Assumptions are bad. You ask the questions, you ask how it affects you...you ask, don't assume.

The idea of therapists asking their clients about their experiences and what they need was something that Chloe brought up several times throughout our discussion, and she continued that theme when talking further about intersectionality:

> You could be the most professional of professionals on that par-ticular subject, but that person's still going to have a different expe-rience to every other person you've met. Because it isn't the same. It's a spectrum. They're all spectrum disorders. That's the reason. And I also find that often every condition somehow connects, and it may not be very direct, it may simply be that I get pain, pain causes anxiety, yeah. Or when I'm "POTSy," that causes pain, which causes anxiety. A bit of a cycle of everything kind of happens and it's just, you don't just get one thing; you somehow get all of it. And one other thing is, if the doctors understand that whoever it is, if they say that they have a really good read of how they feel, there's a really good chance that they do that, they do really know how they're feeling in their body and can really read what's happening where, and the doctors need to listen to that because they don't know what that person's feeling. They're not experiencing it.

> And if the client says that they're in a lot of pain, then yes. The doctor needs to listen. And, like, if I say I'm in a lot of pain, can you

do something about it? Like, is there any way we can help with this? The doctor needs to listen, and you know, go, "Well we can do this or we can do this." Or, "I understand that you're probably in a lot of pain. I'm really sorry you have to be experiencing that."

Chloe also mentioned the importance of acknowledging a client's experiences again:

> Yeah. Acknowledging that you're in a lot of pain. It feels good to be acknowledged and feels good to go hear someone say, "Yeah, you're in pain. I'm sorry you have to be dealing with that, but here we can do something to help with it." Because that's a good thing to hear.

> It's also always great when you hear "We can do something to help with your pain or can do something to help with your anxiety." That's good in general if you don't have to be feeling this.

SOCIAL SKILLS

Finally, I asked Chloe how she felt about neurodivergent children or teens being taught social skills:

> I don't have strong opinions. But I think that if neurodivergent kids are going to be taught how to fit in with neurotypical people, neurotypical people should also be taught how neurodivergent people work because it shouldn't just be the one way. Neurodivergent people have to learn how to fit in with neurotypical people because we have to "be the same as them." Like, I feel like that's a bit of my opinion on what social skills is. It very much also depends on how you do it. You have to be very mindful of, it's not about making the kids fit in, it's about helping them feel comfortable...not making them fit in.

Because it never should be about fitting in. It should be about feeling comfortable. And that's why I believe that neurotypical people should also be taught how neurodivergent people work. Because goodness, all the neurodivergent people are being taught about everything neurotypical people do and exactly how to fit in with the neurotypical people. But most of those neurotypical people have no idea what neurodivergence is. So, like, if we're going to force neurodivergent people to fit in with society, society should just be able to adapt to them. And anyone who dare say that neurodivergent people are very stuck and stubborn and can't change their ways are very wrong and has no idea what neurodiversity is.

Goodness. We change everything about ourselves just to fit in. We do a lot to fit in with neurotypical people. So, I believe that if we're going to do that much, neurotypical people should at least consider doing something for us. And making it easier for us rather than forcing us to change everything to hide our feelings. So, teaching social skills is something...you do it not to teach them how to fit in, but teach them how to feel comfortable.

Making neurodivergent people feel comfortable rather than making them fit in was a repeated part of Chloe's response, which is exactly what the neurodiversity affirming framework is about. So I asked Chloe how she thought we could support neurodivergent children and adolescents to feel comfortable in social situations:

Sometimes it can be as simple as just doing a group with other kids, other neurodivergent kids, other neurotypical kids. It can just be doing stuff with other kids and being part of something and getting involved in something. It doesn't have to be focused on learning exactly how to socialize. It can just be doing something like doing a Minecraft session together and, in that, going, how comfortable are you with talking to people? Let's get out of our comfort zones a bit and try and really communicate and have a bit of fun together. And rather than really focusing on communicating, like trying to fit in with the narrative world, just having neurodivergent kids get comfortable with being around other kids and talking with other kids...that can make a lot more of a difference.

I wondered why neurodivergent children don't necessarily feel safe and comfortable socializing, and what Chloe thought about that:

It's not that... I'm not really saying that that's a thing that all neurodivergent kids get, but I know that I definitely struggle with socialization. If, like, doing all the socializing groups that I did, I think a lot of them were very focused on learning how to communicate. Yeah. Neurotypically. Like, they were very much an open space, but I feel, like, if we were just given the opportunity to socialize with each other, which I feel, like, that's actually kind of what we did, that's something that I find would be much more helpful. Like, personally, because I struggle a lot with socializing, I find that I would much rather just do a group with someone, do Dungeons and Dragons or something like that and just build that confidence because it's harder to become confident when you don't want to communicate with people. I think it's hard for neurodivergent people. I think it'd just be a good thing in general having socializing groups.

Given Chloe's experience with groups, and her personal challenges socializing, I asked Chloe whether she felt like some people might have difficulty because they've had negative experiences previously trying to socialize with people, and so they learn not to put themselves in social situations:

I would say absolutely. Yeah. Because one thing with neurodivergent people is they often will say exactly what they're thinking, and in the neurotypical world that can be very offensive. If those kids who struggled with that, they're probably not wanting to communicate with other people because they think they're doing something wrong. And that's why they probably need a place to communicate with other kids and learn that they're not doing anything wrong. It's just the other kids don't get it.

Something that really stood out for me in Chloe's responses was the impact that we, as clinicians, have on our client's experiences, and the importance of trust, listening, and collaboration. It also seemed very clear in our discussions that being neurodiversity affirming doesn't have to be difficult. There are many simple ways to show a client that you accept, value, and care about them.

I'm so grateful to Chloe for her willingness to share her experiences. I think there is an enormous amount that we can learn from Chloe about how we can best support our child and adolescent clients. I hope you found Chloe's insights as valuable as I have.

Chapter 15

Emotional Identification, Expression, and Regulation

Differences in the identification, expression, and regulation of emotions are associated with many types of neurodivergence, and are frequently linked to challenges reported by parents and educators with regard to a child's social skills and behaviors of concern. These differences have also fed persistent myths, such as that Autistic individuals lack empathy and are not interested in friendships, an idea that has been disproven time and time again but that continues to be brought up by individuals who lack insight and understanding into neurodivergence.

To be very clear, neurodivergent individuals *do* experience emotions and *do* have empathy, although there are differences in the way neurodivergent individuals process, perceive, and express emotions that are often misunderstood or misinterpreted by the neurotypical community.

EMOTIONAL IDENTIFICATION

While some neurodivergent individuals are very good at identifying feelings and have a good insight into the feelings of others (leading some of us to become psychologists!), others have significant difficulty in this area.

Some neurodivergent children will find it difficult to recognize emotions in themselves due to challenges with interoception. As mentioned in Chapter 11, interoception is the sense that tells us what is happening in our bodies, and it is closely linked to our understanding and regulation of emotions. Most neurotypical individuals will notice changes in their body that occur when they feel different emotions. For example, children might feel energized when excited, hot when angry, or breathless when scared. Children might also experience an increased heart rate when angry, or nausea when worried. Many neurodivergent children have difficulty noticing and understanding these messages in their bodies, which can make it challenging for them to recognize what emotion they may be experiencing.

In my clinical work, I have seen many neurodivergent children who experience high levels of anxiety every day, but when I have spoken to them about the emotions they experience, they say that they only feel happy or angry. The situations the children describe as making them feel angry are often situations in which other children might indicate feeling sad, scared, or worried as well as angry, but these children only report angry feelings. It is as if they can distinguish between what might be seen as positive and negative emotions, but are not able to identify more specific emotional states within each category. It is often not until we have worked out ways to reduce their anxiety that they start to recognize and perhaps really feel other emotions, but before that it is almost as if the anxious feelings are so strong, that they drown everything else out.

For other children, their interoception is disorganized and doesn't deliver clear signals, so even though they may know they are feeling something, they have to guess what the feeling is. The discomfort of not knowing how they feel can in itself result in anxiety and distress.

Neurodivergent individuals who have difficulty identifying their feelings may also struggle with labeling their feelings with words. It could be challenging for them to say how they might be feeling if a particular situation occurs, or how they felt when something happened in the past, as well as having difficulty using words to describe their feeling in the moment. For some of my clients, coming up with their own words to describe how they feel in certain situations can help them and others better understand their experiences. Words might be a combination of traditional feelings words that seem to suit the emotion the child is experiencing (e.g., "nercited," a combination of excited and nervous), or a completely different word that has meaning for them (e.g., "struggly," when they are uncomfortable, stressed, and dysregulated).

With regard to recognizing feelings in others, neurodivergent children can sometimes have difficulty reading neurotypical facial expressions and body language to determine what someone is feeling. This may be due to difficulty recognizing emotions in themselves, and therefore finding it hard to identify feelings in others, as they don't have the vocabulary or level of understanding of how others might feel in different situations. This may also be compounded by the tendency for neurotypical individuals to say one thing but mean something different (e.g., saying things like "I'm fine" when they look angry or upset).

It is important to remember that there will be considerable variation between the emotion identification skills of neurodivergent individuals, and assumptions should not be made one way or the other with regards to where an individual's skills might be. I have met a number of neurodivergent children who had rote-learned what physical symptoms they were expected to have when experiencing different feelings and when these feelings might occur, but actually did not personally relate to any of these in real life, and so while they could recite what they had learned, it wasn't meaningful or useful for them. For example, when asked about how their body feels when they are worried, they reported that their heart beats fast and their stomach feels sick. But when we discussed specific situations where they felt worried, they reported that they did not notice anything changing in their body until they had gone into meltdown. We need to work together with neurodivergent children and adolescents and be curious about their experiences to determine whether they are having difficulty in this area and how we can best assist them.

EMOTIONAL EXPRESSION

For neurodivergent individuals, particularly those who are Autistic or ADHDers, differences in emotional expression are often highlighted as significant challenges. For example, neurodivergent children may be described as having facial expressions and body language that are flat and difficult to read, or have their emotional responses being classed as inappropriate and excessive by neurotypical individuals. The problem with these observations of neurodivergent emotional expression is that they are extremely subjective and are based on neurotypical expectations.

As mentioned in Chapter 2, the "double empathy problem," introduced as a concept by Dr. Damian Milton, goes a long way to explaining the difficulty neurotypical and neurodivergent individuals have in interpreting each other's emotional expression and social communication. It is not that one way is right and the other is wrong; it's that due to what could be seen as cultural differences, it is difficult to clearly or confidently interpret and understand the feelings of each other. This can be rectified by each individual taking the time to understand the other person's emotional expression. However, while much time is spent teaching neurodivergent children about neurotypical emotional expression, little time is spent on the reverse.

When working from a neurodiversity affirming framework, it is essential that children understand that all feelings are okay—there are no right or wrong feelings in any given situation, and generally, no right or wrong way to express those feelings. Particularly for Autistics and ADHDers, I find that they are often taught about feelings in terms of positive and negative, and are frequently reprimanded for their emotional reactions to situations, leading to them feeling ashamed of their feelings and thinking there is something wrong with them for having a big response to a situation or getting angry or upset. Children need to be taught that all feelings are valid and have a purpose, and we don't have to change a feeling or feel bad for having it. If feelings are acknowledged as natural and meaningful for the individual, and their expression is explored and understood from the perspective of the child, rather than feeling ashamed, children can learn to listen to their emotions and work with them.

It is important to honor an individual child's way of expressing their emotions, and for those caring for them to learn to read the signals the child is giving to determine how they feel. There should be no difference between a child smiling and laughing when they are happy and a child jumping and flapping when they are happy. Just because a feeling is being expressed in a different way doesn't make it wrong. Further, what does it matter if someone is very expressive in their facial expressions and body language, or alternatively quite neutral or serious? I think the reason that neurotypical individuals have highlighted the idea of "flat affect" so much, especially with Autistic individuals, is that it makes them feel uncomfortable to not be able to tell how someone feels. But it shouldn't be about their comfort; it should be about allowing everyone to express themselves in their own way.

When supporting children to understand emotions, it is important that we provide examples of the many ways emotions may be expressed, and highlight possible similarities and differences between emotional expression in neurotypical and neurodivergent individuals. This supports children to develop an understanding of their own emotions as well as learning to read and interpret the expressions of others.

EMOTIONAL REGULATION

Challenges with emotional regulation are certainly one of the most common reasons I have for referral of neurodivergent children at my practice, and I know it is something that many neurodivergent children struggle with.

Neurodivergent children often experience emotions more deeply and intensely than their neurotypical peers, and as such may have more difficulty with regulating their emotional responses, both positive and negative. I often hear parents say that their neurodivergent child is fairly neutral in their expression of emotion most of the time, when they are going about their daily routines, but when a situation elicits a big emotion, such as happy, sad, or angry, they express it in what might be considered an extreme way. It is like an emotion can pass over a neurodivergent child like a huge wave that is all-consuming in the moment, and then it is gone. This may be why some parents report frustration in their child becoming extremely upset about something at home, and crying and screaming about it for an extended period of time, and then they calm down and move on like nothing happened, while the parent is still dealing with all the residual feelings they have about the situation.

When supporting neurodivergent children with emotional regulation challenges, it is obviously important that they can identify and understand their emotions before they are able to regulate or manage them, so that is where we, as clinicians, need to start.

Exploring whether a child has an awareness and understanding of interoception is really important when working with children on emotional regulation, as we often support children to look for physical warning signs that they are becoming frustrated, overwhelmed, or anxious, and these signs usually involve interoception. If the child does not have clear signals from their body, they may be unable to notice any warning signs. Indeed, some of my clients tell me that they don't notice any changes in their body until they are in full meltdown, and then it is too late for them to use any strategies to calm or regulate. For children who struggle with interoception, I have found that supporting them to notice external behavior signs can be helpful for them, as well as working on building their interoceptive awareness in the longer term.

I think it is also very important within a neurodiversity affirming framework to help children understand what is happening in the brain and body when they are experiencing emotions, and particularly when their stress response is activated. Learning about how their brain is wired to respond to stress and challenging situations, and that a person's "thinking brain" and "feeling brain" don't communicate well with each other when someone is distressed, can be really powerful in supporting them to understand why they sometimes feel out of control, and what they might be able to do to help themselves get through these situations better.

For most children, what they can do to manage better is actually preventative rather than something they should do in the moment. It is about learning to look after themselves and manage their energy levels and stress throughout the day to help them to stay regulated.

Depending on the age of the child, it can be helpful to use an analogy like a battery, or a character's "health points" in a game, to talk about what things in their day take their energy and what things give them energy back, so they can start to understand the need for balance. For younger children this is something that is important for parents to understand and support their children with, because they will not be able to do it alone.

Teaching relaxation and calming techniques such as mindfulness and meditation, and supporting children to identify their own activities that make them feel calm, are also important elements of supporting children with emotional regulation. Exploring different activities to find those that work for each individual child will be necessary, as some children will find breathing and visualization helpful, whereas others may prefer to listen to music, or perhaps do some coloring or drawing. These techniques may be helpful for children to use if they identify they are becoming upset or heightened, but are also great for a child to engage in regularly to support their overall wellbeing.

You might have guessed by now that emotional regulation is linked closely with sensory sensitivities, arousal, and regulation, which we discussed earlier, in Chapters 6, 8, and 11. Sensory input can lead to emotional regulation challenges in children and can also certainly be a powerful tool in supporting neurodivergent children to regulate. Autism Level UP! has some great resources available to support emotional regulation and arousal. A link to their website can be found in the "Useful Resources" section at the end of the book.

Something that I think is important to mention when discussing emotional regulation is the idea of the "size of the problem." Many emotional literacy programs teach children that they should consider how big a problem is, or how important the issue is, and match their reaction to whatever size the problem is perceived to be. The biggest issue with this is that it invalidates the child's experience of the situation and the feelings they have about it, and their response would be considered wrong if it doesn't match an arbitrary rating of the problem by neurotypical standards. For example, if an adult deems the problem of an iPad running out of battery as a small problem, but it is very upsetting to the child and they cry and scream, then the child would be said to have had the incorrect or an inappropriate response.

This method of teaching about emotional regulation also does not take into account anything else that is impacting on the child and their response; the behavior is just labeled as not matching the size of the problem, and as such needs to be changed. This does not fit within neurodiversity affirming practice.

To be neurodiversity affirming with regard to emotional regulation, we need to validate and acknowledge the child's perception of the situation and the feeling they are having, and work with them to resolve the problem. Now obviously, if a child is hurting themselves or others when they experience big feelings, we will want to support them to find a safer way to do this, but this doesn't negate the feeling the child is having or how big it is; it is about finding ways to express this that keeps everyone safe.

Finally, when we are supporting a child with emotional regulation, it is absolutely essential that we consider the child's developmental level and their capacity to self-regulate. It is common for young children to attend therapy with goals centered around emotional regulation that involve them learning calming or regulating strategies and using them independently. However, what these types of goal fail to recognize is that children learn to self-regulate through co-regulation, and as such, they will likely continue to need some adult support to regulate their arousal and manage big feelings until they are approaching their preteen years.

SOME OTHER TOPICS OF NOTE REGARDING EMOTIONS

Co-regulation

Co-regulation can be defined as another individual, usually a caring adult, using their presence and own arousal level to support a child to manage big feelings and regulate their arousal level. Parents do this with babies all the time, holding them and supporting them to calm with their presence, but we often forget that children still need this support, although it may look different.

While parents may still use their physical presence to co-regulate through a hug or perhaps lying next to a younger child, with older children they may just sit next to them or be in the room but a short distance away. The key is that they are present with them and supporting them to regulate by meeting their dysregulation and heightened or distressed state with calm. This might involve speaking quietly to them; it might involve breathing slowly with them; it might involve just being there. But a calming presence will have an impact on their nervous system through mirror neurons, and bring their arousal level closer to where the parents are.

This is important for parents to know, but it is equally important for us, as clinicians, to recognize and to use to support our clients. If a client comes into a session dysregulated, we can use our presence to support them through co-regulation. If they are heightened, we may initially meet them part way and be more elevated with them in our energy level, and then gradually bring ourselves down to a more regulated state, and hopefully bring them down too.

It is important to note that this can also work in the opposite way. If we go into a session heightened or stressed due to anticipation of a difficult session or perhaps something unrelated but challenging happening before we start, we may inadvertently elevate our client's arousal level and lead to both the client and ourselves becoming dysregulated.

Sometimes it can be helpful to describe what is happening for you at the same time as regulating yourself, noticing out loud that you are feeling a bit dysregulated, or whatever word works for your client, and then modeling breathing or stretching or doing a quiet activity to regulate, and inviting them to join you.

Hyper empathy

We have already discussed the double empathy problem and established that neurodivergent children do, in fact, have empathy, but I wanted to briefly also bring the concept of hyper empathy to your attention, as it is something that does impact on some members of the neurodivergent community.

The concept of hyper empathy really comes from the idea that some individuals can be extremely empathic and sensitive to other people's emotions. This is thought to be a kind of synesthesia, when the brain and body interpret one kind of sensory information in another modality.

Where this can become particularly challenging for neurodivergent children (and adults) is that it can be difficult to separate the individual's own emotions from the emotions of the people around them. This can have a significant impact on the neurodivergent individual as they are often experiencing amplified negative or difficult emotions, which can be extremely draining and distressing. In addition, the neurodivergent individual's reaction can easily be misinterpreted by those around them. For example, an Autistic child might see a friend fall over and hurt their knee in the playground and start to cry. The Autistic child feels their friend's distress intensely, and immediately starts to cry as well. Usually what happens in these situations is that the Autistic child is told off for trying to take attention away from the hurt child or to stop being silly, and their behavior is interpreted as a lack of empathy when it is, in fact, the opposite.

As clinicians, recognizing that hyper empathy can occur and being curious about our clients' experiences can lead to a greater understanding for the client and ourselves, and open up other ways to talk about emotional experiences.

Meltdowns and shutdowns

Meltdowns and shutdowns are unfortunately quite a common experience for neurodivergent individuals, and cause a significant amount of distress to the child and often the people around them.

Meltdowns and shutdowns occur when a neurodivergent individual's brain and nervous system are triggered into survival mode and a "fight, flight, or freeze" response. Meltdowns and shutdowns can be triggered by a range of factors, including sensory or cognitive overload, anxiety or stress, past trauma, intense emotions, or sudden change.

When working from a neurodiversity affirming perspective, we recognize that when a child is in meltdown or shutdown, they are on autopilot and acting to keep themselves safe. As such, they do not have control of their words and actions. Further, the most effective way to support a child in meltdown or shutdown is to ride the wave and co-regulate if you can. The goal during a meltdown is to keep everyone safe until it is over, and then to support the child to calm and regulate.

Staying safe may look different depending on your setting and where the child is, but it usually involves remaining in the room with a child but at a safe distance (if possible), keeping talking to a minimum, reducing eye contact, and perhaps sitting down to make yourself less threatening. For some children, talking about a special interest or something you enjoy doing together can assist with regulating and distracting, but it will depend on the child and how well you know them. It is important not to put your hands on the child or try and take things off them unless there is a serious safety risk (e.g., a child trying to jump out of a window). As soon as you touch a child in an elevated state, you are much more likely to be injured and also risk re-traumatizing the child if they have had a similar experience before.

Enlisting the support of a parent or colleague is definitely advisable in these situations—remembering that the goal is to keep everyone safe and to wait it out.

Given that the child is not in control of their actions during a meltdown or shutdown, it is extremely important that a child is not punished or penalized in any way for anything they did while dysregulated and out of control. This means that we do not ask for an apology, or make a child clean up any mess they have made; we just want to support them to calm. If an opportunity arises in which you can talk to the child when they are calm, about what made them upset or triggered the meltdown or shutdown and what you could do to support them next time, that can be helpful. Alternatively, you may want to just reflect and debrief with a colleague about what occurred and what you can do to reduce the likelihood of the child becoming distressed next time you see them.

If you would like more information about supporting children and adolescents in meltdown and without restraint, please see the link to Studio 3 in the "Useful Resources" section at the end of the book.

— Chapter 16 —

Social Skills

Many neurodivergent neurotypes have historically been associated with social skills difficulties, and as such, social skills training has been a considerable focus of therapy for neurodivergent children, particularly those identified as Autistic, ADHD, or with Learning Disabilities.

In recent years, there has been a change in the direction of social skills training to support neurodivergent individuals to better understand their own way of socializing and communicating, and to help them understand how neurotypical individuals engage in social interaction, rather than trying to teach neurodivergent individuals to act in neurotypical ways.

Knowledge from adults sharing their lived experience, theories such as the double empathy problem, and research into neurodivergent communication and social interaction has paved the way for these changes, as evidence for differences in social communication and interaction rather than deficits has pushed us to rethink our understanding of social interaction and what is involved.

Underlying all the discussions and changes in thinking around this area is the question "Is there a right and a wrong way to socialize?" For years we have operated on the premise that social skills are black and white, and the neurotypical way of socializing is right, while other ways of socializing are wrong. This has resulted in neurodivergent children being taught that they must interact with others according to neurotypical social rules if they are to be successful in connecting and forming relationships (e.g., making eye contact, taking turns when talking, keeping your body still when listening, greeting people with a smile and a wave, etc.), and all the while there has been little interest from the neurotypical population to meet neurodivergent children half-way and to try and understand their way of doing things because it was just viewed as wrong.

With an understanding of neurodiversity affirming practice comes a realization that we have been sending neurodivergent children a message for years that they are wrong, that they are faulty, that they are broken, because they don't do things the way neurotypical people do. What we need to be doing instead is celebrating the culture of neurodivergence and the richness of the differences that this culture brings to our community. We should not expect neurodivergent children to follow neurotypical conventions or judge their interactions and behaviors by neurotypical standards.

We need to remove the burden of effective social interaction being solely on the neurodivergent individual. The double empathy problem highlights this by suggesting that the social disconnect that is often present between neurotypical and neurodivergent individuals is due to both parties having different social styles and difficulty understanding each other due to those differences.

There are now social skills curriculums being designed for school classrooms that celebrate neurodiversity and teach all students about the different ways that we communicate and socialize. This is the direction in which we need to head if we want to see real change— neurotypical children need to be supported to understand and be accepting of neurodivergent ways of doing things too.

In the meantime, teaching neurodivergent children about social communication and interaction looks different from a neurodiversity affirming perspective.

To begin with, we need to support neurodivergent clients to understand that there are many different ways of engaging in social communication and interaction. We can do this by providing examples of a range of social behaviors that we might see in interactions with others, and then discussing what they notice themselves doing, and perhaps what they notice friends or peers doing too.

We might then support a client to understand in general the social style of neurodivergent individuals and the social style of neurotypical individuals and the similarities and differences between them. This can be a good time to introduce the concept of perspective-taking and exploring how a client feels when their social partner does and says certain things, and what their partner may think and feel about what your client does and says based on the different social expectations of neurotypical individuals compared with neurodivergent individuals.

Notice that at no point in these discussions have we talked about one way of doing things being better than another, or the "right" way. We are just talking about differences. The important part of teaching a child about social skills in this way is that they can then choose how to interact with peers and friends in social situations. It also gives them the tools to advocate for themselves with their friends if their social style is being misinterpreted. For example, a neurodivergent child might choose to ask a neurotypical friend questions when they are sharing a story about something because they recognize that their neurotypical friend sees this as showing interest and it makes them feel good. Alternatively, a neurodivergent child might explain to a neurotypical friend that they find it hard to stay still and look at them while they are listening, but they are definitely paying attention and want to hear what their friend has to say.

I often still hear clinicians saying things like "but the child is coming home crying about not having friends and wants to learn how to make them." And then this is used as a justification for teaching a child explicit neurotypical social skills. The main problem with this is that we are teaching the child to mask and pretend to be someone else in order to fit in, which has repercussions for their ongoing mental health. Also, the reality is that many neurodivergent children who do try to use neurotypical social skills they have learned explicitly in therapy are not very successful and end up not being accepted anyway. In a situation like this, where a child is struggling to make friends and is feeling sad about this, it is better to advocate for the child to have opportunities to socialize with other children, perhaps in interest groups where they will meet like-minded children, and support them to understand that they will find people who accept them for who they are and that is better than pretending so people will like them. Providing opportunities for a child to build their confidence in socializing with others is also important if the child has had numerous experiences of being rejected or left out, and I find interest groups are a great way to do this.

When thinking about social skills, another factor to consider is why social skills have come up as a focus for a child. This will often be brought up by parents who are worried that their child does not have friends, or perhaps only has one good friend, and they feel like they need help to connect with others so they will be happier. It is really important in these situations to check in with the child about what friendship looks like for them, and whether it is important to them or not. For some neurodivergent children, it might be more important for them to feel like they belong rather than having individual friends, and so being part of a larger group of children, and sitting and listening to their interactions, might be what makes them happy. Other children might really want to connect with someone and be able to talk to them or play with them. Others still may not feel the need to socialize at all, and might be happy to speak with children in class but prefer to take time for themselves at recess and lunch. When we are being neurodiversity affirming, none of these options are wrong; they are just different and suited to each individual child.

Something that does come up in conversations about friendships, particularly for adolescents, is online friends. Many neurotypical individuals seem to have an opinion that online friendships are not real because you don't really know the individual or meet with them in person. However, this is, again, placing neurotypical standards on neurodivergent experiences.

If we think about what neurotypical individuals usually look for in friendships, it would probably be things like talking to each other regularly, hanging out and perhaps gaming or playing sport together, having shared interests, having a laugh together, and with closer friends, perhaps sharing personal experiences and getting advice. While many of these things might usually be done in person, they can also all be done online. Why is that less meaningful?

Of course, we need to make sure that children and teens are safe online, so teaching about cyber safety and monitoring their online communication is important, and restricting communication with unknown individuals on public sites is essential. However, there are now many reputable and moderated ways for neurodivergent children and teens to connect with peers online, and also games that allow parents to restrict access only to children who are known to the child (e.g., from school) that can open up a neurodivergent child's or adolescent's social world.

Another situation I see occurring often is the pathologizing of neurodivergent friendships in situations that wouldn't be considered a concern for neurotypical children. For example, when an Autistic child has one close friend, you may hear clinicians and educators saying that the child needs to be supported to branch out and be with other people to form more connections. Then the Autistic child and their friend are placed in separate classrooms the following year to encourage this change. However, if a neurotypical child has one close friend it is usually considered "normal" and nothing is said or done about it. Often taking action is justified by well-meaning adults who are concerned that if the neurodivergent child's one friend is away, they won't have anyone else to play with, or they want the child to learn to make other friends because they will have to do it when they go to high school or go to work. But we don't put neurotypical children through this. As clinicians, we need to resist the urge of some parents and educators to therapize every minute of a neurodivergent child's life, so they are learning or practicing skills, and instead let them have time to do their own thing and find their own way, offering support only if and when the need arises.

Supporting neurodivergent children and adolescents to socialize and connect with peers in their own way, while also developing an understanding of how neurotypical socializing works, sets them up to have positive social experiences and to find peers who will accept them for who they are.

Chapter 17

Self-Care and Independence

Being able to care for yourself and be independent in life are goals that most of us strive to achieve, and for neurodivergent individuals, this is no exception. However, taking a neurodiversity affirming approach to self-care and independence means supporting children to develop self-care skills that are functional and useful for them to improve their independence and quality of life in areas that they are motivated to make change, not trying to force them to learn skills that will make other people's lives easier. It is also about acknowledging aspects of their lives that they may always struggle with, and finding ways to accommodate those challenges.

I find that parents can often get caught up in a child having skills that they will possibly need as adults, and be in a hurry for them to be able to do things on their own, when the reality is that developmentally they may not yet be able to master these skills. In addition to this, children may have sensory sensitivities, anxiety, and executive functioning challenges that are barriers to them participating in activities required for personal hygiene and self-care, leading to considerable frustration for families and the children themselves when they are unable to do things they feel they should, or that they see their peers doing.

A classic example of this that occurs in many families is the child who is physically capable of getting dressed themselves, but who does not have the executive function in terms of organization, concentration, and working memory to complete the task on their own. These are the children who have their uniform laid out on the bed for them and are told to get dressed, the parent leaves the room to get a sibling ready, and when they come back five minutes later the child is sitting on the floor in their underwear playing with LEGO®. The result is frustration for the parent, and confusion and often shame for the child who gets into trouble every morning for not getting dressed, but just can't seem to do it no matter how hard they try. The point is that it is not about trying harder; it is about actually having the skill necessary to do the task. Despite perhaps knowing how to do it, the child is clearly not yet actually ready to get dressed on their own; they need their parent to be there with them, talking through what to put on next, or handing them their clothes. Ultimately, it will be quicker and less stressful for everyone to stay with the child and work with them to get dressed than to keep coming back and forth to the child and finding they have not completed the task. It is not about what the child "should" be able to do; it is meeting them where they are, and providing the support necessary to assist them to have success.

As a neurodiversity affirming therapist, it is important to support clients and families to understand what skills are reasonable to expect from a developmental and disability perspective, and how these skills can be gradually built up over time with support and opportunities. It is important to present accommodations that can be used both until a skill is acquired and as an ongoing support if the skill is something that may not be possible to acquire fully and will always involve some level of assistance or modification. I find that in many settings, particularly at times of transition such as a child moving from primary school to secondary or high school, there is a sudden push for children to be independent so they can cope with increased expectations likely to be placed on their skills and behavior. Unfortunately, in my experience this often means schools or parents removing the child's existing supports so they can supposedly learn to do things themselves because "they won't have someone helping them when they get to high school!" or "they need to learn how to function in the real world." My response to this is "Why? Why won't a child have access to supports they need when they are older? Do they suddenly stop having a disability? And what is so wrong with needing help in the first place?"

I believe that part of our role as neurodiversity affirming clinicians is to normalize this need for supports at home, at school, and out in the community, at whatever level the individual needs as they grow and develop. As discussed in Chapter 4, we need to be presuming competence and providing opportunities with supports in place to allow children to achieve and participate. The reality is that complete independence is a myth. We all need other people and different tools to allow us to function day to day, and there is nothing wrong with that. In fact, it allows us all to do better than we might otherwise.

I would like to note here that the need for support for any individual varies greatly, and for individuals with high support needs, access to the necessary supports can actually be a matter of life or death. As clinicians, we need to recognize the caring role that families provide, and also the intensive assistance that is necessary to allow individuals with high support needs to access everyday activities, and advocate for clients and families to have the level of support necessary to allow them to live full and satisfying lives.

With regard to self-care activities such as washing, eating, and toileting, it is essential to work with the child and family to encourage skill development and support the implementation of accommodations. It is important to ensure that the child's rights as a human being are being honored in any intervention that is embarked on, as well as taking into consideration sensory sensitivities, anxiety, and other needs. I say this particularly in relation to self-care, although it is obviously also important in any other way you are working with a child, because in most self-care activities a child's bodily autonomy comes into question. I am aware of clinicians who continue to encourage the forced feeding or forced washing of children, and even punishment for toileting accidents or being unable to swallow certain foods, which is only going to lead to a child experiencing potential trauma and a damaged relationship with their parent. While a child does need to wash to ensure they do not get sores or skin infections, and certainly a child must eat and drink to stay alive, being neurodiversity affirming means taking the child's individual needs into consideration and working with them and their family to find ways to support them in a safe and respectful way that allows growth in their own time.

For example, for a child with a very limited diet, this may mean suggesting to a parent that they cook chicken nuggets and chips for dinner every night, and have some other foods available at the table with no pressure to try them or not. It may mean working on hand strength and coordination to use cutlery in therapy, but allowing a child to eat mostly finger food at home to ensure they eat enough without becoming fatigued or frustrated. Perhaps it will mean the addition of a supplement to ensure they get the vitamins and minerals they need, or allowing them to eat frozen peas straight from the freezer or covering their meals with tomato sauce. As clinicians we need to move past trying to make a neurodivergent child eat in a neurotypical way, and adjust our expectations and our recommendations to ensure success for the child and family.

Many families will, understandably, focus on striving for neurotypical standards when it comes to their child's self-care and daily routine. For example, there is an expectation that everyone should sit and eat a meal together at dinner time, that everyone should shower or bath daily, and that teeth should be brushed twice a day. There are also often rules about things like what food should be eaten at certain times (e.g., cereal is a breakfast food), how much screentime a child should have, when children should go to bed, and how a child should hold their pencil to write. While some of these expectations may come from cultural expectations that are important to families, and as such we need to try and work within them, many expectations are based on nothing more than it being the way everyone does it, and so there is implicit pressure for families of neurodivergent children to do it too.

In many ways, I think it is part of our role as clinicians to give families permission or approval to do things differently, because for many of our families there is an inbuilt fear of judgment about going against the norm. Being neurodiversity affirming involves looking at the child and family's unique situation, and supporting them to find what works for them.

— Chapter 18 —

Speech and Language

We have already discussed the need to honor neurodivergent communication in therapy (see Chapter 4), but how can clinicians be neurodiversity affirming in the support of language and communication development in children? The answer is not so much what skills are being taught, but how they are being taught.

Neurodivergent children, just like neurotypical children, may present with conditions that impact on their ability to communicate, such as Verbal Apraxia, expressive and receptive language disorders, articulation challenges, or stuttering. Depending on their challenges, children may benefit from support to improve articulation and fluency, develop speech sounds and vocabulary, understand language, or communicate using AAC.

I think the most important focus for speech pathology, particularly for young children, is to support them to find ways to communicate effectively in whatever way works for them. If they already have speech but they are difficult to understand, then articulation work would likely be appropriate. If they do not have any spoken language, then working on speech sounds may be appropriate, but it would also be essential to explore other ways for the child to communicate using AAC at the same time. All children should have an opportunity to learn to communicate their needs in the easiest and most effective way possible.

It is not considered neurodiversity affirming to wait to see whether a child develops some spoken language over 6–12 months before introducing alternate means of communication. Waiting like this denies a child the opportunity to have their voice heard. Further, research suggests that the use of AAC does not reduce or negatively impact speech development, so introducing alternate ways to communicate is not going to stop a child talking if they are able. What it is going to do is reduce frustration in the child, and assist them to have their needs understood and met.

As I mentioned earlier (see Chapter 4), the actual focus of speech therapy is generally not an issue, but the way speech therapy is conducted can be problematic if therapists take a behavioral approach. For example, in the past, some speech therapists, using methods that were considered "best practice" at the time, may have withheld items until a child spoke a word or made a sound to request them. Or perhaps they removed a child's AAC device to try and encourage the child to speak. This style of working is compliance-based and does not respect the child's autonomy or communication preference.

To be neurodiversity affirming, clinicians need to work with the child's strengths and interests, and provide opportunities for modeling and practicing target skills through play, games, and activities that the child enjoys or finds meaningful. If a child does not want to do something, clinicians need to honor that choice. It is our job as therapists to find something else that the child wants to do, and to try and incorporate therapy goals into that.

At no time in therapy should a child's mode of communication be taken away or made unavailable. Taking away a child's AAC is essentially taping the child's mouth shut, which, of course, we would never do to a child who can speak, so it is essential that a child has access to their device at all times. If they choose not to use it at any point, it is their choice, and that should be respected.

Beyond basic communication and vocabulary development, neurodivergent children are often taken to a speech and language pathologist or psychologist to develop their social communication or pragmatic language skills. Traditionally this has involved teaching children neurotypical social rules such as how to take turns in a conversation, how to show interest and be a good listener, how to stay on topic, and how not to offend people by bluntly telling them the truth.

As we have already discussed in relation to social skills, what neurodivergent children need is support to understand the way that they communicate and how that might differ from their neurotypical peers, rather than being taught that they do things wrong and that they need to learn to do it right. For example, an ADHDer may learn that they tend to interrupt and talk over others because when they think of something to say they want to say it before they forget, whereas neurotypical individuals will usually wait until there is a break in a conversation before saying something. Or an Autistic child may learn that their style of communicating involves info-dumping or sharing lots of information about a topic of interest with friends, whereas neurotypical individuals tend to like taking turns to talk by sharing smaller pieces of information and asking questions or commenting to show interest.

These differences also extend to non-verbal communication or body language, with eye contact in particular being the source of much controversy in recent years. Eye contact has been widely taught as an essential element of communication, and has been forced onto neurodivergent children by neurotypical adults in countless ways in the past, including children having their head held and forcibly turned to face an adult, or the endlessly repeated refrain "Look at me while I'm talking to you!" We now know that eye contact is at best a discomfort and at worst painful to many neurodivergent individuals, particularly Autistics, and as such should not be taught or required by clinicians in neurodivergent communication.

It is important for neurodivergent children to understand their own communication style and that of their neurotypical peers, to allow them to navigate social situations effectively. However, we are not teaching them to change their communication style to fit in. We are supporting them to understand that neurotypical individuals like to communicate in a particular way, and so there may be things that we do and say that they may misunderstand, or the other way round.

One thing that I do teach neurodivergent children to do where possible is to ask for clarification when they are unsure of what someone means or how they are feeling, rather than remaining unclear about whether they are interpreting a neurotypical peer's language and behavior accurately or not. This is a way that they can be proactive in managing a social situation effectively.

Finally, when appropriate, it is important to support children to develop the language around advocating for themselves and their needs (as discussed in Chapter 13). This is something that doesn't just involve language, but also confidence and an insight into their neurodivergence. It can be an incredibly empowering process for a child to go through, and can support them to be upfront and open with friends and family about their needs and the way they do things in the hope that understanding will lead to acceptance. For example, an Autistic teen may be able to say to their friends something like "When I get excited about something I can keep talking about it forever. If I've been talking for ages and you want to say something, just say 'Sally, can I say something?' and I will stop and listen." This way, the friends are finding ways to both have their needs met while still honoring their individual communication styles.

Supporting communication in neurodiversity affirming ways is not just providing neurodivergent children and adolescents with a voice, but also giving them the tools to be successful in the social world without having to sacrifice who they are.

— Chapter 19 —

Play

According to the World Health Organization, having access to play is a child's basic human right, and we are continually advancing in our understanding of the importance of play and how it benefits child development. However, just as other parts of child development have traditionally focused on neurotypical patterns, so, too, has the area of play.

The definition of play is one that varies considerably in the research, and there are many different types of play that have been described by child development experts and researchers over the last few decades. However, there is general consensus of a number of play types seen in child development, including exploratory play, sensory play, construction play, motor play, cause and effect play, functional play, and pretend or imaginative play.

Play by definition is child-led, open-ended, and enjoyable or fun, which would suggest that there is no right way to play. However, play differences in neurodivergent children have been pathologized over many years, resulting in a focus on intervention programs aimed at teaching pretend play skills.

The reason that pretend play appears to be the main focus of interventions is that differences in the development of pretend play are evident in some neurodivergent populations (e.g., Autistic individuals), and research has linked pretend play skills, which typically develop fully by around five years of age in neurotypical children, with the later development of problem-solving, literacy, and language skills. The research, however, is not conclusive in neurodivergent populations, and focuses on observable behaviors in play rather than internal processes, so children may be engaging in pretend play but may not be doing it in a clearly observable way, and are therefore assumed to be engaged in an alternate play behavior.

For example, an Autistic child may spend time setting up a dolls house with furniture and placing the figures in specific places and then move on to another activity. It may appear to an observer that the child has merely organized the toys and then left them; however, the child may have created an elaborate story in their head while arranging the toys and has moved on because the story is finished. So they may have engaged in pretend play, but to some observers it simply doesn't look like it.

Unfortunately, rather than being allowed to play in their own way and have their preferences and choices respected, many neurodivergent children have their play interrupted and structured by adults in an effort to build neurotypical play skills. This, in turn, sends the message once again that there is something wrong with the child and how they do things, and that they need to learn to do it differently to fit in. It could also be argued that once an adult intervenes and changes what the child is doing, it is no longer technically play, as it is not in the child's control.

To be neurodiversity affirming with regard to play, we need to take the neurodivergent child's lead and allow them to engage in activities their way. It is also important not to apply neurotypical standards to neurodivergent play, as the motivations and internal processes involved may be very different to how things appear on the surface. An example of this is the idea of social play, which, from a neurotypical perspective, would usually involve children playing together collaboratively and interacting together. For neurodivergent children, however, social play may occur more in parallel, with children alongside each other playing their own games but commenting or sharing the experience with each other. As parallel play is considered a lesser form of play than cooperative or collaborative play by neurotypical standards, the neurodivergent children would be considered less developed and potentially in need of intervention, when there is nothing wrong with how they are playing and interacting.

It is also important to remember that there are benefits for children in engaging in all kinds of play. For example, sensory play (e.g., playing with water, sand, slime, Play-Doh, rice, smells, sounds, etc.) is known to support brain development and neuronal connection, assist with sensory processing, and support arousal regulation, as well as also being beneficial to the development of problem-solving and language skills. Sensory play is also seen to be an essential part of the process of healing for children who have experienced trauma early in life, as it supports the development of connection between a child's "survival" brain and other higher order brain structures. This assists a child to move out of a mostly hypervigilant state to a more regulated state in which they are less likely to be triggered into a stress response.

Given that many neurodivergent children are hypervigilant to threat and have a heightened stress response, it makes sense to me that they may seek out sensory play more often than neurotypical children, and may continue with sensory play after their neurotypical peers have moved on to other types of play, because their brain and sensory system needs it. Unfortunately, because sensory play tends to be a focus of younger neurotypical children, and is then often passed over for more social and pretend play as children get older, neurodivergent children are often discouraged from this type of play, and pushed to engage in the "more advanced" neurotypical play of their peers.

Research into the benefits of play has identified what are known as the "Therapeutic Powers of Play," a list of 20 processes that are thought to be agents of change in social-emotional development and healing through play. According to Charles Schaefer and Athena Drewes, both experts in the field of play therapy, these agents of change can facilitate communication, foster emotional wellness, increase personal strengths, and enhance social relationships. As clinicians, we do not need to teach a child how to play in order to utilize these therapeutic benefits; we can join a child in their play, and connect with them on their terms.

We need to allow neurodivergent children to have autonomy in their play choices and play the way they need and want to play, whether that be solitary or social, pretend, sensory, or any other type of play, so they can benefit from these processes and develop their play skills at their own pace and in their own way.

— Chapter 20 —

A Final Reflection

So, you've made it to the end of the book and your head is swimming with ideas and strategies and things you might want or need to change.

But now what?

How can you possibly implement all of the things described in this book with your clients? It's just not possible! Or is it?

Well, I have good news for you... You don't have to do it all at once.

As I said early in the book, neurodiversity affirming practice is a philosophy, not a set of rules to follow.

You now have greater awareness and understanding of what being neurodiversity affirming means and why it is important, and that knowledge will guide you as you move forward and start to make changes in the way you engage your clients and their families.

You might have some long-held habits that you will need to try and break, like using person-first language.

You might want to try some things out and see if they actually make a difference, because you're not totally convinced.

You might want to start with just one thing—perhaps writing neurodiversity affirming goals—and then see how things go after that.

You might just start noticing all the things you already do that are neurodiversity affirming, and reflect on that.

It doesn't matter how you start or what you do first, as long as you give it a try.

And please remember that even when it feels like second nature, there will be times when you won't get it right. And that's okay, too.

Every change you make, however small, is likely to lead to another change, and then another. And those changes will really make a difference to the lives of your clients and their families.

So thank you again for reading this book, and good luck!

Useful Resources

MORE ABOUT NEURODIVERSITY AFFIRMING PRACTICE

Autism Level UP!: www.autismlevelup.com

Autism Spectrum News: https://autismspectrumnews.org

Autistic Self Advocacy Network (ASAN): https://autisticadvocacy.org

NeuroClastic: https://neuroclastic.com

Neurodiversity Hub: www.neurodiversityhub.org

Reframing Autism: https://reframingautism.org.au

Therapist Neurodiversity Collective: https://therapistndc.org

LIVED EXPERIENCE EXPERTS

Yael Clark, Developmental Psychologist: https://supportingparents.com.au

Rachel Dorsey, Autistic SLP: https://dorseyslp.com/aboutme

Raelene Dundon: https://raelenedundon.com

Kristy Forbes, Intune pathways: www.kristyforbes.com.au

Emily Hammond, NeuroWild: www.facebook.com/profile.php?id=100087870753308

Cynthia Kim, Musings of an Aspie: https://musingsofanaspie.com/essential-reading

Emily Lees, Autistic SLP: www.autisticslt.com

Jessica McCabe, How to ADHD: https://howtoadhd.com

Sandhya Menon, Onwards & Upwards Psychology: www.onwardsandupwardspsychology.com.au

Neurodivergent Doctor: https://neurodivergentdr.wixsite.com/website

Mrs. Speechie P: www.mrsspeechiep.com

Dr. Nick Walker, Neuroqueer: https://neuroqueer.com

NEURODIVERSITY AFFIRMING ALLIES

Dr. Mona Delahooke: https://monadelahooke.com

Bo Hejlskov Elvén: https://eng.hejlskov.se

Jessie Ginsburg, MS, CCC-SLP: www.jessieginsburg.com

Dr. Ross Greene, Originator of the Collaborative & Proactive Solutions Approach: https://drrossgreene.com/index.htm; www.cpsconnection.com/skill-enhancement-parents

Libby Hill, Small Talk Speech Therapy: www.smalltalkspeechtherapy.com.au/blog

Kelly Mahler, Interoception Groupie and Occupational Therapist: www.kelly-mahler.com

Professor Andrew McDonnell, *The Reflective Journey* book: www. studio3.org/product-page/the-reflective-journal

Dr. Bruce Perry and Beacon House: www.bdperry.com; https://beaconhouse.org.uk/resources

Greg Santucci, Occupational Therapist: https://gregsantucci.com

Dr. Stuart Shanker, The MEHRIT Centre: https://self-reg.ca

Dr. Dan Siegel: https://drdansiegel.com

Studio3: www.studio3.org

Dr. Peter Vermeulen, Autism in Context: https://petervermeulen.be

Bibliography

PART 1: IN THEORY

Chapter 1, What Is Neurodiversity?

American Psychiatric Association (2013) *Diagnostic and Statistical Manual of Mental Disorders, Fifth Edition*. Philadelphia, PA.

Armstrong, T. (2010) *Neurodiversity: Discovering the Extraordinary Gifts of Autism, ADHD, Dyslexia, and Other Brain Differences*. Boston, MA: Da Capo Press.

Armstrong, T. (2011) *The Power of Neurodiversity: Unleashing the Advantages of Your Differently Wired Brain*. Boston, MA: Da Capo Lifelong Books.

Armstrong, T. (2020) "The cultural context of neurodiversity." American Institute for Learning and Human Development, January 24. Accessed on January 28, 2023, from www.institute4learning.com/2020/01/24/the-cultural-context-of-neurodiversity

Chapman, R. (2020) "Defining Neurodiversity for Research and Practice." In H. B. Rosqvist, N. Chown and A. Stenning (eds) *Neurodiversity Studies: A New Critical Paradigm*. Abingdon: Routledge.

Chapman, R. (2021) "Negotiating the neurodiversity concept." *Psychology Today, Australia*, August 18. Accessed on January 20, 2023, from www.psychologytoday.com/au/blog/neurodiverse-age/202108/negotiating-the-neurodiversity-concept

Gonzalez, M., Saxena, S., Chowdhury, F., Dyck Holzinger, S., Martens, R., Oskoui, M., and Shikako-Thomas, K. (2022) "Informing the development of the Canadian Neurodiversity Platform: What is important to parents of children with neurodevelopmental disabilities?" *Child: Care, Health and Development 48*, 1, 88–98. https://doi.org/10.1111/cch.12906

Lost in my Mind TARDIS (no date) "PSA from the actual coiner of 'neurodivergent'." Accessed on January 20, 2023, from https://sher-locksflataffect.tumblr.com/post/121295972384/psa-from-the-actual-coiner-of-neurodivergent

Singer, J. (2017) *Neurodiversity: The Birth of an Idea*. Self-published, Kindle Edition.

Stenning, A. and Rosqvist, H. B. (2021) "Neurodiversity studies: Mapping out possibilities of a new critical paradigm." *Disability & Society 36*, 9, 1532–1537. https://doi.org/10.1080/09687599.2021.1919503

Walker, N. (no date) "Neurodiversity: Some basic terms & definitions." Neuroqueer. Accessed on January 20, 2023, from https://neuroqueer.com/neurodiversity-terms-and-definitions

Chapter 2, What Does It Mean to Be Neurodiversity Affirming?

ASAN (Autistic Self Advocacy Network) (no date) "Identity-first language." Accessed on January 29, 2023, from https://autisticadvocacy.org/about-asan/identity-first-language

Bottema-Beutel, K., Kapp, S. K., Lester, J. N., Sasson, N. J., and Hand, B. N. (2021) "Avoiding ableist language: Suggestions for Autism researchers." *Autism in Adulthood*, 18–29. http://doi.org/10.1089/aut.2020.0014

Brown, D. (2021) "Neurodiversity-affirming care." Video podcast, April 10. Accessed on January 29, 2023, from https://affectautism.com/2021/04/10/neurodiversity

den Houting, J. (no date) "Why everything you know about autism is wrong." TEDxMacquarieUniversity, TED Talk. Accessed on January 20, 2023, from www.ted.com/talks/jac_den_houting_why_everything_you_know_about_autism_is_wrong?language=en

Gernsbacher, M. A. (2017) "Editorial Perspective: The use of person-first language in scholarly writing may accentuate stigma." *The Journal of Child Psychology and Psychiatry 58*, 7, 859–861. https://doi.org/10.1111/JCPP.12706

Goering, S. (2015) "Rethinking disability: The social model of disability and chronic disease." *Current Reviews in Musculoskeletal Medicine 8*, 2, 134–138. https://doi.org/10.1007/S12178-015-9273-Z

Kornblau, B. L. and Robertson, S. M. (2021) "Special issue on occupational therapy with neurodivergent people." *American Journal of Occupational Therapy 75*, 3. https://doi.org/10.5014/AJOT.2021.753001

Milton, D. E. M. (2012) "On the ontological status of autism: The 'double empathy problem'." *Disability & Society 27*, 6, 883–887. https://doi.org/1 0.1080/09687599.2012.710008

Milton, D. (2018) "The double empathy problem." National Autistic Society, March 2. Accessed on January 20, 2023, from www.autism.org.uk/ advice-and-guidance/professional-practice/double-empathy

Taboas, A., Doepke, K., and Zimmerman, C. (2022) "Short report: Preferences for identity-first versus person-first language in a US sample of autism stakeholders." *Autism 27*, 2. https://doi.org/10.1177/13623613221130845

Watson, S. and Constantino, C. D. (2022) "Autistic is me: As the movement to embrace an autistic identity—and resist neuro-normative pressure and ableism—gathers steam, what are the implications for professional practice?" *The ASHA Leader 27*, 3, 12–20. Accessed on February 22, 2023, from https://leader.pubs.asha.org/do/10.1044/leader.FTR1.27052022. ableism-autism.12/full

Chapter 3, Why Are Changes in Therapeutic Practice Needed?

Arstein-Kerslake, A., Maker, Y., Flynn, E., Ward, O., Bell, R., and Degener, T. (2020) "Introducing a human rights-based disability research methodology." *Human Rights Law Review 20*, 3, 412–432. https://doi.org/10.1093/ hrlr/ngaa021

Melnyk, B. M., Fineout-Overholt, E., Stillwell, S. B., and Williamson, K. M. (2010) "Evidence-based practice: Step by step: The seven steps of evidence-based practice." *The American Journal of Nursing 110*, 1, 51–53, from https://journals.lww.com/ajnonline/Fulltext/2010/01000/Evi- dence_Based_Practice__Step_by_Step__The_Seven.30.aspx

Olson, J. D. M. (2021) *Implementing Evidence-Based Practice*. CINAHL Nursing Guide.

Reynolds, J. M. (2017) "'I'd rather be dead than disabled'—the ableist con- flation and the meanings of disability." *Review of Communication 17*, 3, 149–163. https://doi.org/10.1080/15358593.2017.1331255

Rogoff, B., Dahl, A., and Callanan, M. (2018) "The importance of understanding children's lived experience." *Developmental Review 50*, 5–15. https://doi.org/10.1016/J.DR.2018.05.006

Sabatello, M., Burke, T. B., McDonald, K. E., and Appelbaum, P. S. (2020) "Disability, ethics, and health care in the COVID-19 pandemic." *American Journal of Public Health 110*, 10, 1523–1527. https://doi.org/10.2105/AJPH.2020.305837

Subramaniam, A. (2021) "Why lived experience matters." *Psychology Today, Australia*, September 29. Accessed on January 29, 2023, from www.psychologytoday.com/au/blog/parenting-neuroscience-perspective/202109/why-lived-experience-matters

University of South Australia (no date) "Guides | Evidence-Based Practice | Overview." Accessed on January 29, 2023, from https://guides.library.unisa.edu.au/ebp/Overview

Vanaken, G.-J. (2022) "Cripping vulnerability: A disability bioethics approach to the case of early autism interventions." *Tijdschrift voor Genderstudies 25*, 1, 19–40. https://doi.org/10.5117/TVGN2022.1.002.VANA

Chapter 4, What Are the Principles of Neurodiversity Affirming Practice?

Armstrong, T. (2020) "Exploring the cultural context of neurodiversity." American Institute for Learning and Human Development, January 24. Accessed on January 28, 2023, from www.institute4learning.com/2020/01/24/the-cultural-context-of-neurodiversity

AssistiveWare (no date) "Gestalt language processing and AAC." Accessed on January 20, 2023, from www.assistiveware.com/blog/gestalt-language-processing-aac

Baird, L. (2022) "Transforming allied health: The 'how' of neurodiversity-affirming services." Reframing Autism, March 17. Accessed on January 29, 2023, from https://reframingautism.org.au/transforming-allied-health-the-how-of-neurodiversity-affirming-services

Brown, H. M., Stahmer, A. C., Dwyer, P., and Rivera, S. (2021) "Changing the story: How diagnosticians can support a neurodiversity perspective from the start." *Autism: The International Journal of Research & Practice 25*, 5, 1171–1174. https://doi.org/10.1177/13623613211001012

Dallman, A. R., Williams, K. L., & Villa, L. (2022) "Neurodiversity-affirming practices are a moral imperative for occupational therapy." *The Open Journal of Occupational Therapy 10*, 2, 1–9. https://doi. org/10.15453/2168-6408.1937

DeThorne, L. S. and Gerlach-Houck, H. (2023) "Resisting ableism in school-based speech-language therapy: An invitation to change." *Language, Speech & Hearing Services in Schools 54*, 1, 1–7. https://doi. org/10.1044/2022_LSHSS-22-00139

Edelstein, R. (2022) "Cultural learning & cultural special education: A different way of thinking about neurodiversity." Different Brains, August 13. Accessed on January 28, 2023, from https://differentbrains.org/cultural-learning-cultural-special-education-a-different-way-of-thinking-about-neurodiversity

Gillespie-Lynch, K., Kapp, S. K., Shane-Simpson, C., Smith, D. S., and Hutman, T. (2014) "Intersections between the autism spectrum and the internet: Perceived benefits and preferred functions of computer-mediated communication." *Intellectual and Developmental Disabilities 52*, 6, 456–469. https://doi.org/10.1352/1934-9556-52.6.456

Gobbo, K. and Shmulsky, S. (2020) "Should neurodiversity culture influence how instructors teach?" *Academic Exchange Quarterly 23*, 4.

Hein, I. M., de Vries, M. C., Troost, P. W., Meynen, G., van Goudoever, J. B., and Lindauer, R. J. L. (2015) "Informed consent instead of assent is appropriate in children from the age of twelve: Policy implications of new findings on children's competence to consent to clinical research ethics in public health, medical law, and health policy." *BMC Medical Ethics 16*, 1, 1–7, from https://link.springer.com/article/10.1186/s12910-015-0067-z

leonardoyeates (2019) "Autistic communication differences & how to adjust for them." NeuroClastic, June 9. Accessed on January 29, 2023, from https://neuroclastic.com/autism-autistic-communication-differences/?fbclid=IwAR3YpxSba7AUjLKH3ihtV4ezMizjwSY2DZooFC4pQ3uJp-Jh3CYVb7-gsUrQ

Pingree, C. A. (no date) "What does presumed competence mean?" Carmen B. Pingree Autism Center. Accessed on January 20, 2023, from https:// carmenbpingree.com/blog/what-does-presumed-competence-mean

Rosenzweig, R. and Prizant, B. M. (2022) "Guidelines for a more neurodiversity-affirming practice for autism." *Autism Spectrum News*, April 1.

Accessed on January 29, 2023, from https://autismspectrumnews.org/guidelines-for-a-more-neurodiversity-affirming-practice-for-autism

Stout, A. (no date) "Presuming competence: What is it and why is it important?" The Autism Site News. Accessed on January 20, 2023, from https://blog.theautismsite.greatergood.com/presume-competence

The People Practice (no date) "Create a strengths-based culture and embrace neurodiversity in the workplace." Accessed on January 28, 2023, from https://thepeoplepractice.com.au/blog/create-a-strengths-based-culture-and-embrace-neurodiversity-in-the-workplace

Chapter 5, Which Therapy Approaches Are Considered Neurodiversity Affirming?

Cooper, K., Loades, M. E., and Russell, A. (2018) "Adapting psychological therapies for autism." *Research in Autism Spectrum Disorders 45*, 4–50, from https://www.sciencedirect.com/science/article/abs/pii/S175094671730123X

Department of Defense (2020) *The Department of Defense Comprehensive Autism Care Demonstration, Annual Report 2020*. Washington, DC.

Dickson, K. S., Lind, T., Jobin, A., Kinnear, M., Lok, H., and Brookman-Frazee, L. (2021) "A systematic review of mental health interventions for ASD: Characterizing interventions, intervention adaptations, and implementation outcomes." *Administration and Policy in Mental Health and Mental Health Services Research 48*, 857–883. https://doi.org/10.1007/s10488-021-01133-7

Ekman, E. and Hiltunen, A. J. (2015) "Modified CBT using visualization for autism spectrum disorder (ASD), anxiety and avoidance behaviour: A quasi-experimental open pilot study." *Scandinavian Journal of Psychology 56*, 6, 641–648. https://doi.org/10.1111/sjop.12255

Gitimoghaddam, M., Chichkine, N., McArthur, L., Sangha, S. S., and Symington, V. (2022) "Applied behavior analysis in children and youth with autism spectrum disorders: A scoping review." *Perspectives on Behavior Science 45*, 3, 521–557, from https://link.springer.com/article/10.1007/s40614-022-00338-x

Goodyear-Brown, P. (2009) *Play Therapy with Traumatized Children*. New York: John Wiley & Sons Inc.

Hillman, H. (2018) "Child-centered play therapy as an intervention for children with autism: A literature review." *International Journal of Play Therapy 27*, 4, 198–204. https://doi.org/10.1037/pla0000083

Kidd, T. (2022) *Helping Autistic Teens to Manage Their Anxiety: Strategies and Worksheets Using CBT, DBT, and ACT Skills*, London: Jessica Kingsley Publishers.

Lobregt-van Buuren, E., Sizoo, B., Mevissen, L., and de Jongh, A. (2019) "Eye Movement Desensitization and Reprocessing (EMDR) therapy as a feasible and potential effective treatment for adults with Autism Spectrum Disorder (ASD) and a history of adverse events." *Journal of Autism and Developmental Disorders 49*, 151–164. https://doi.org/10.1007/s10803-018-3687-6

Lowry, M. (no date) "What is autistic-centered therapy?" Accessed on January 29, 2023, from www.mattlowrylpp.com/blog/act-83tka

Malchiodi, C. (2014) *Creative Interventions with Traumatized Children*, Second Edition (Creative Arts and Play Therapy series). New York: Guilford Press.

Sandoval-Norton, A. H., Shkedy, G., and Shkedy, D. (2019) "How much compliance is too much compliance: Is long-term ABA therapy abuse?" *Cogent Psychology 6*, 1, from https://www.researchgate.net/publication/334377318_How_Much_Compliance_is_Too_Much_Compliance_Is_Long-Term_ABA_Therapy_Abuse

Schottelkorb, A. A., Swan, K. L., and Ogawa, Y. (2020) "Intensive child-centered play therapy for children on the autism spectrum: A pilot study." *Journal of Counseling & Development 98*, 1, 63–73. https://doi.org/10.1002/jcad.12300

Shkedy, G., Shkedy, D., and Sandoval-Norton, A. H. (2019) "Treating self-injurious behaviors in autism spectrum disorder." *Cogent Psychology 6*, 1, from https://www.tandfonline.com/doi/full/10.1080/23311908.2019.1682766

Wise, S. J. (2022) *The Neurodivergent Friendly Workbook of DBT Skills: A Workbook of Dialectical Behaviour Therapy Skills Reframed to Be Neurodivergent Friendly with the Added Bonus of Accessible Mindfulness Practices, Sensory Strategies and Managing Meltdowns.* Lived Experience Educator.

Wood, J. J., Drahota, A., Sze, K., Har, K., Chiu, A., and Langer, D. A. (2009) "Cognitive behavioural therapy for anxiety in children with autism spectrum disorders: A randomized, controlled trial." *Journal of Child*

Psychology and Psychiatry 50, 3, 224–234, from https://www.ncbi.nlm. nih.gov/pmc/articles/PMC4231198/

PART 2: IN PRINCIPLE

Chapter 6, The Therapeutic Relationship

Ardito, R. B. and Rabellino D. (2011) "Therapeutic alliance and outcome of psychotherapy: Historical excursus, measurements, and prospects for research." *Frontiers in Psychology 2*, 270, from https://www.ncbi.nlm.nih. gov/pmc/articles/PMC3198542/ PMID: 22028698; PMCID: PMC3198542.

Bozarth, J. D. (2013) "Unconditional Positive Regard." In M. Cooper, M. O'Hara, P. E. Schmid, and A. C. Bohart (eds) *The Handbook of Person-Centred Psychotherapy & Counselling* (pp.180–192). London, New York, Dublin: Bloomsbury Academic.

Cherry, K. (2020) "Unconditional positive regard in psychology." Very Well Mind, May 10. Accessed on January 20, 2023, from www.verywellmind. com/what-is-unconditional-positive-regard-2796005

Dodson, W. W. (2016) "Emotional regulation and rejection sensitivity." Accessed on March 24, from https://chadd.org/wp-content/ uploads/2016/10/ATTN_10_16_EmotionalRegulation.pdf

Farber, B. A., Suzuki, J. Y., and Ort, D. (2022) "What Is Positive Regard, and Why Is It Important?" In B. A. Farber, J. Y. Suzuki, and D. Ort (eds) *Understanding and Enhancing Positive Regard in Psychotherapy: Carl Rogers and Beyond*. American Psychological Association. https://doi. org/10.1037/0000312-002

Follette, W. C., Naugle, A. E., and Callaghan, G. M. (1996) "A radical behavioral understanding of the therapeutic relationship in effecting change." *Behavior Therapy 27*, 4, 623–641.

Kossak, M. S. (2009) "Therapeutic attunement: A transpersonal view of expressive arts therapy." *The Arts in Psychotherapy 36*, 1, 13–18. https:// doi.org/10.1016/j.aip.2008.09.003

Norcross, J. C. (2010) "The Therapeutic Relationship." In B. L. Duncan, S. D. Miller, B. E. Wampold, and M. A. Hubble (eds) *The Heart and Soul of Change: Delivering What Works in Therapy* (pp.113–141). Philadelphia, PA: American Psychological Association. https://doi.org/10.1037/12075-004

Chapter 7, Goal-Setting

Costa, U. M., Brauchle, G., and Kennedy-Behr, A. (2017) "Collaborative goal setting with and for children as part of therapeutic intervention." *Disability and Rehabilitation 39*, 16, 1589–1600. https://doi.org/10.1080/09 638288.2016.1202334

Dawson, G., Franz, L., and Brandsen, S. (2022) "At a crossroads—Reconsidering the goals of autism early behavioral intervention from a neurodiversity perspective." *JAMA Pediatrics 176*, 9, 839–840. https://doi.org/10.1001/jamapediatrics.2022.2299

Dorsey, R. (no date) "Goal writing for autistic students." Accessed on January 29, 2023, from https://dorseyslp.com/blog/goalwritingfor autisticstudentsblog

Gore, K. (2021) "How to avoid writing ableist goals in speech therapy." speech IRL, February 23. Accessed on January 29, 2023, from www.speechirl.com/how-to-avoid-writing-ableist-goals-in-speech-therapy

Levine, S. L., Holding, A. C., Milyavskaya, M., Powers, T. A., and Koestner, R. (2021) "Collaborative autonomy: The dynamic relations between personal goal autonomy and perceived autonomy support in emerging adulthood results in positive affect and goal progress." *Motivation Science 7*, 2, 145–152. https://doi.org/10.1037/mot0000209

Pritchard, L., Phelan, S., McKillop, A., and Andersen, J. (2020) "Child, parent, and clinician experiences with a child-driven goal setting approach in paediatric rehabilitation." *Disability and Rehabilitation 44*, 7, 1042–1049. https://doi.org/10.1080/09638288.2020.1788178

Roberts, J. (2020) "On writing masking goals for autistic middle school girls—Stop it!" Therapist Neurodiversity Collective, August 13. Accessed on February 22, 2023 from https://therapistndc.org/masking-goals-autistic-middle-school-girls

Chapter 8, Sensory Differences and Regulation

Dunn, W. (2007) "Supporting children to participate successfully in everyday life by using sensory processing knowledge." *Infants & Young Children 20*, 2, 84–101, from https://journals.lww.com/iycjournal/Fulltext/2007/04000/ Supporting_Children_to_Participate_Successfully_in.2.aspx

Kapp, S. K., Steward, R., Crane, L., Elliott, D., Elphick, C., Pellicano, E., and Russell, G. (2019) "'People should be allowed to do what they like': Autistic adults' views and experiences of stimming." *Autism: The*

International Journal of Research & Practice 23, 7, 1782–1792. https://doi.org/10.1177/1362361319829628

Mayer, J. L. (2017) "The relationship between autistic traits and atypical sensory functioning in neurotypical and ASD adults: A spectrum approach." *Journal of Autism and Developmental Disorders 47*, 2, 316–327.

Metz, A. E., Boling, D., DeVore, A., Holladay, H., Liao, J. F., and Vlutch, K. V. (2019) "Dunn's model of sensory processing: An investigation of the axes of the four-quadrant model in healthy adults." *Brain Sciences 9*, 2, 35. DOI: 10.3390/brainsci9020035.

Miller, L. J., Schoen, S. A., Mulligan, S., and Sullivan, J. (2017) "Identification of sensory processing and integration symptom clusters: A preliminary study." *Occupational Therapy International*, 2876080, from https://www.ncbi.nlm.nih.gov/pmc/articles/PMC5733937/

Tsuji, Y., Matsumoto, S., Saito, A., Imaizumi, S., Yamazaki, Y., Kobayashi, T., Fujiwara, Y., Omori, M., and Sugawara, M. (2022) "Mediating role of sensory differences in the relationship between autistic traits and internalizing problems." *BMC Psychology 10*, 148. https://doi.org/10.1186/s40359-022-00854-0

Chapter 9, Reframing Behavior

Delahooke, M. (2019) *Beyond Behaviors: Using Brain Science and Compassion to Understand and Solve Children's Behavioral Challenges*. Eau Claire, WI: Pesi Inc.

Elven, B. H. and Wiman, T. (2017) *Sulky, Rowdy, Rude? Why Kids Really Act Out and What to Do About It*. London: Jessica Kingsley Publishers.

Greene, R. W. (2011) *The Explosive Child*. London: HarperCollins Publishers Ltd.

Hughes, D. and Golding, K. (2012) *Creating Loving Attachments: Parenting with Pace to Nurture Confidence and Security in the Troubled Child*. London: Jessica Kingsley Publishers.

Kohn, A. (2018) *Punished by Rewards: The Trouble with Gold Stars, Incentive Plans, A's, Praise, and Other Bribes*. Twenty-fifth Anniversary Edition. London: HarperOne.

McDonnell, A. (2019) *The Reflective Journey: A Practitioner's Guide to the Low Arousal Approach*. Alcester: Studio3.

McDonnell, A. and Deveau, R. (2018) "Low arousal approaches to manage behaviours of concern." *Learning Disability Practice 21*, 5, 30–36. https://doi.org/10.7748/LDP.2018.E1882

Perry, B. D. and Winfrey, O. (2021) *What Happened to You? Conversations on Trauma, Resilience, and Healing*. New York: Flatiron Books.

Shanker, S. and Barker, T. (2016) *Self-Reg: How to Help Your Child (and You) Break the Stress Cycle and Successfully Engage with Life*. New York: Penguin Press.

Woodcock, L. and Page, A. (2010) *Managing Family Meltdown: The Low Arousal Approach and Autism*. London: Jessica Kingsley Publishers.

Chapter 10, Masking

Barnes, M. (2022) "Masking: What is it and why do neurodivergent people do it?" Psychreg, September 13. Accessed on January 29, 2023, from www.psychreg.org/masking-what-why-neurodivergent-people-do-it

Bernardin, C. J., Mason, E., Lewis, T., and Kanne, S. (2021) "'You must become a chameleon to survive': Adolescent experiences of camouflaging." *Journal of Autism and Developmental Disorders 51*, 12, 4422–4435. https://doi.org/10.1007/S10803-021-04912-1

Cage, E. and Troxell-Whitman, Z. (2019) "Understanding the reasons, contexts and costs of camouflaging for autistic adults." *Journal of Autism and Developmental Disorders 49*, 5, 1899–1911. https://doi.org/10.1007/S10803-018-03878-X

McQuaid, G. A., Lee, N. R., and Wallace, G. L. (2021) "Camouflaging in autism spectrum disorder: Examining the roles of sex, gender identity, and diagnostic timing." *Autism 26*, 2, 552–559. https://doi.org/10.1177/13623613211042131

Perry, E., Mandy, W., Hull, L., and Cage, E. (2022) "Understanding camouflaging as a response to autism-related stigma: A social identity theory approach." *Journal of Autism and Developmental Disorders 52*, 2, 800–810. https://doi.org/10.1007/s10803-021-04987-w

Petrolini, V., Rodríguez-Armendariz, E., and Vicente, A. (2023) "Autistic camouflaging across the spectrum." *New Ideas in Psychology 68*. https://doi.org/10.1016/j.newideapsych.2022.100992

Wood-Downie, H., Wong, B., Kovshoff, H., Mandy, W., Hull, L., and Hadwin, J. A. (2021) "Sex/gender differences in camouflaging in children and adolescents with autism." *Journal of Autism and Developmental Disorders* *51*, 4, 1353–1364. https://doi.org/10.1007/s10803-020-04615-z

Chapter 11, Intersectionality

American Academy of Allergy Asthma & Immunology (no date) "Mast Cell Activation Syndrome (MCAS)." Accessed on January 20, 2023, from www.aaaai.org/conditions-treatments/related-conditions/mcas

Botha, M. and Frost, D. M. (2020) "Extending the minority stress model to understand mental health problems experienced by the autistic population." *Society and Mental Health 10*, 1, 20–34. https://doi.org/10.1177/2156869318804297

Csecs, J., Iodice, V., Rae, C. L., Brooke, A., Simmons, R., Quadt, L., Savage, G. K., Dowell, N. G., Prowse, F., Themelis, K., Mathias, C. J., Critchley, H. D., and Eccles, J. A. (2022) "Joint hypermobility links neurodivergence to dysautonomia and pain." Hypermobility Syndromes Association, October 27. Accessed on January 20, 2023, from www.hypermobility.org/post/joint-hypermobility-links-neurodivergence-to-dysautonomia-and-pain

De Thierry, B. (2016) *The Simple Guide to Child Trauma: What It Is and How to Help* (Simple Guides). London: Jessica Kingsley Publishers.

Dysautonomia International (no date) "What is dysautonomia?" Accessed on January 20, 2023, from www.dysautonomiainternational.org/page.php?ID=34

Farquhar-Leicester, A. L., Tebbe, E., and Scheel, M. (2022) "The intersection of transgender and gender-diverse identity and neurodiversity among college students: An exploration of minority stress." *Psychology of Sexual Orientation and Gender Diversity.*

Giupponi, G., Giordano, G., Maniscalco, I., Erbuto, D., Berardelli, I., Conca, A., Lester, D., Girardi, P., and Pompili, M. (2018) "Suicide risk in attention-deficit/hyperactivity disorder." *Psychiatria Danubina 30*, 1, 2–10, from https://www.researchgate.net/publication/323783187_Suicide_risk_in_attention-deficithyperactivity_disorder

Glidden, D., Bouman, W. P., Jones, B. A., and Arcelus, J. (2016) "Gender dysphoria and autism spectrum disorder: A systematic review of the literature." *Sexual Medicine Reviews 4*, 1, 3–14. https://doi.org/10.1016/j.sxmr.2015.10.003

Gould, Z. (2022) "Somewhere under the double rainbow—Discussing LGBTQAI+ and neurodiversity intersectionality." Social Care Institute

for Excellence, June 29. Accessed on January 20, 2023, from www.scie.
org.uk/tackling-inequality/blogs/pride-zoe

Gray-Hammond, D. (2020) "Autism, ADHD, Tourette's, dyslexia: Higher
risk for addiction & suicide- #NoDejahVu." NeuroClastic, September
9. Accessed on January 20, 2023, from https://neuroclastic.com/neu-
rodivergent-people-are-more-at-risk-of-suicide-and-addiction-speak-
up-nodejahvu

Green, M. (2020) "Neurodiversity: What is it and what does it look
like across races?" OpenLearn, Open University, September 8.
Accessed on January 20, 2023, from www.open.edu/openlearn/
health-sports-psychology/mental-health/neurodiversity-what-
it-and-what-does-it-look-across-races

Kirby, A. V., Bakian, A. V., Zhang, Y., Bilder, D. A., Keeshin, B. R., and Coon,
H. (2019) "A 20-year study of suicide death in a statewide autism pop-
ulation." *Autism Research: Official Journal of the International Society for
Autism Research 12*, 4, 658–666. https://doi.org/10.1002/aur.2076

Livingston, E. M., Siegel, L. S., and Ribary, U. (2018) "Developmental
dyslexia: Emotional impact and consequences." *Australian Journal of
Learning Difficulties 23*, 2, 107–135, from https://www.researchgate.net/
publication/325907379_Developmental_dyslexia_emotional_impact_
and_consequences

Lyons, S., Whyte, K., Stephens, R., and Townsend, H. (2020) "Developmental trauma close up." Beacon House. Accessed on January 29,
2023, from https://beaconhouse.org.uk/wp-content/uploads/2020/02/
Developmental-Trauma-Close-Up-Revised-Jan-2020.pdf

Miller, H. L., Thomi, M., Patterson, R. M., and Nandy, K. (2022) "Effects of
intersectionality along the pathway to diagnosis for autistic children
with and without co-occurring attention deficit hyperactivity disorder in
a nationally-representative sample." *Journal of Autism and Developmental
Disorders*, 1–16. https://doi.org/10.1007/s10803-022-05604-0

Moore, I., Morgan, G., Welham, A., and Russell, G. (2022) "The intersection
of autism and gender in the negotiation of identity: A systematic review
and metasynthesis." *Feminism & Psychology 32*, 4, 421–442. https://doi.
org/10.1177/09593535221074806

The Ehlers-Danlos Society (no date) "What is EDS?" Accessed on January
20, 2023, from www.ehlers-danlos.com/what-is-eds

The Trevor Project (2022) "Mental health among autistic LGBTQ youth." April 29. Accessed on January 28, 2023, from www.thetrevorproject.org/research-briefs/mental-health-among-autistic-lgbtq-youth-apr-2022

Wattel, L. L., Walsh, R. J., and Krabbendam, L. (2022) "Theories on the link between autism spectrum conditions and trans gender modality: A systematic review." *Review Journal of Autism and Developmental Disorders*, 1–21. https://doi.org/10.1007/s40489-022-00338-2

Wilmot, A., Pizzey, H., Leitão, S., Hasking, P., and Boyes, M. (2022) "Growing up with dyslexia: Child and parent perspectives on school struggles, self-esteem, and mental health." *Dyslexia: An International Journal of Research and Practice 29*, 1, 40–54. https://doi.org/10.1002/dys.1729

Chapter 12, Supporting and Educating Parents

Armstrong, T. (2011) *The Power of Neurodiversity: Unleashing the Advantages of Your Differently Wired Brain*. Boston, MA: Da Capo Lifelong Books.

Dundon, R. (2017) *Talking with Your Child about Their Autism Diagnosis: A Guide for Parents*. London: Jessica Kingsley Publishers.

Marsh, E. and Heyworth, M. (2022) "Neurodiversity-affirming language: A letter to your family, friends and support network." Reframing Autism, February 14. Accessed on January 30, 2023, from https://reframingautism.org.au/neurodiversity-affirming-language-a-letter-to-your-family-friends-and-support-network

raisingchildren.net.au (no date) "Neurodiversity and neurodivergence: A guide for families." Accessed on January 29, 2023, from https://raisingchildren.net.au/guides/a-z-health-reference/neurodiversity-neurodivergence-guide-for-families

Reframing Autism (2022) "Guidelines for selecting a neurodiversity-affirming mental healthcare provider." Tip sheets and infographics, September 8. Accessed on January 30, 2023, from https://reframingautism.org.au/guidelines-for-selecting-a-neurodiversity-affirming-mental-healthcare-provider

Wright Stein, S., Alexander, R., Mann, J., Schneider, C., Zhang, S., Gibson, B. E., Gabison, S., Jachyra, P., and Mosleh, D. (2022) "Understanding disability in healthcare: Exploring the perceptions of parents of young people with autism spectrum disorder." *Disability and Rehabilitation 44*, 19, 5623–5630.

Chapter 13, Self-Advocacy

Anderson, S. and Bigby, C. (2017) "Self-advocacy as a means to positive identities for people with intellectual disability: 'We just help them, be them really'." *Journal of Applied Research in Intellectual Disabilities 30*, 1, 109–120. https://doi.org/10.1111/jar.12223

Kay, D. (2019) "On the participation of children with medical conditions in risk assessment: A case for development of self-advocacy." *Educational Psychology in Practice 35*, 4, 357–367. https://doi.org/10.1080/02667363.2019.1609424

Leadbitter, K., Buckle, K. L., Ellis, C., and Dekker, M. (2021) "Autistic self-advocacy and the neurodiversity movement: Implications for autism early intervention research and practice. *Frontiers in Psychology 12*, 782, from https://www.ncbi.nlm.nih.gov/pmc/articles/PMC8075160/

Owens, T. L. and Lo, Y. (2021) "Function-based self-advocacy training for students with or at risk for emotional and behavioral disorders in general education settings." *Journal of Emotional and Behavioral Disorders 30*, 3, 185–198. https://doi.org/10.1177/10634266211039760

Rose, M., Chislett, S., Despott, N., Hepburn, J., Johnson, R., and Dawnsong, W. (2020) *Self Advocacy in Healthcare: A Toolkit for LGBTIQA+ Autistic People, Their Family Carers, Friends, Support Workers, and Advocates.* Melbourne: Spectrum Intersections and Inclusion Melbourne.

Tilley, E., Strnadová, I., Danker, J., Walmsley, J., and Loblinzk, J. (2020) "The impact of self-advocacy organizations on the subjective well-being of people with intellectual disabilities: A systematic review of the literature." *Journal of Applied Research in Intellectual Disabilities 33*, 6, 1151–1165. https://doi.org/10.1111/jar.12752

PART 3: IN PRACTICE

Chapter 14, What Do Neurodivergent Children Want from Therapy?

No references for the interview.

Chapter 15, Emotional Identification, Expression, and Regulation

Bennie, M. (2022) "What is alexithymia and its relationship to interoception?" Autism Awareness Centre Inc., September 7. Accessed on January 20, 2023, from https://autismawarenesscentre.com/what-is-alexithymia-and-its-relationship-to-interoception

Delahooke, M. (2019) *Beyond Behaviors: Using Brain Science and Compassion to Understand and Solve Children's Behavioral Challenges*. Eau Claire, WI: Pesi Inc.

Elven, B. and Wiman, T. (2017) *Sulky, Rowdy, Rude? Why Kids Really Act Out and What to Do About It*. London: Jessica Kingsley Publishers.

Goodall, E., Brownlow, C., and Lawson, W. (2022) *Interoception and Regulation: Teaching Skills of Body Awareness and Supporting Connection with Others*. London: Jessica Kingsley Publishers.

Greene, R. W. (2011) *The Explosive Child*. London: HarperCollins Publishers Ltd.

McDonnell, A. (2019) *The Reflective Journey: A Practitioner's Guide to the Low Arousal Approach*. Alcester: Studio3

Palser, E. R., Fotopoulou, A., Pellicano, E., and Kilner, J. M. (2018) "The link between interoceptive processing and anxiety in children diagnosed with autism spectrum disorder: Extending adult findings into a developmental sample." *Biological Psychology 136*, 13–21, from https://www.sciencedirect.com/science/article/pii/S0301051118303235

Shanker, S. and Barker, T. (2016) *Self-Reg: How to Help Your Child (and You) Break the Stress Cycle and Successfully Engage with Life*. New York: Penguin Press.

Woodcock, L. and Page, A. (2010) *Managing Family Meltdown: The Low Arousal Approach and Autism*. London: Jessica Kingsley Publishers.

Chapter 16, Social Skills

Davis, R. and Crompton, C. J. (2021) "What do new findings about social interaction in autistic adults mean for neurodevelopmental research?" *Perspectives on Psychological Science 16*, 3, 649–653. https://doi.org/10.1177/1745691620958010

Dorsey, R. (2020) "The Dilemma of Social Skills Therapy Part 1: The Young Child." Accessed on January 29, 2023, from https://dorseyslp.com/blog/the-dilemma-of-social-skills-therapy

Dundon, R. (2022) "Why social skills training has to go!" January 14. Accessed on January 29, 2023, from https://raelenedundon.com/why-social-skills-training-has-to-go

Morrison, K. E., DeBrabander, K. M., Jones, D. R., Faso, D. J., Ackerman, R. A., and Sasson, N. J. (2020) "Outcomes of real-world social interaction for autistic adults paired with autistic compared to typically developing partners." *Autism 24*, 5, 1067–1080. https://doi.org/10.1177/1362361319892701

Roberts, J. (2021) "Nothing about social skills training is neurodivergence-affirming—Absolutely nothing." Therapist Neurodiversity Collective, May 27. Accessed on January 29, 2023, from https://therapistndc.org/nothing-about-social-skills-training-is-neurodivergence-affirming

White, T. (2022) " How autism may affect social skills." PsychCentral, May 9. Accessed on January 29, 2023, from https://psychcentral.com/autism/autism-social-skills

Chapter 17, Self-Care and Independence

Bailin, A. (2019) "Clearing up some misconceptions about neurodiversity." Scientific American, Observations, June 6. Accessed on January 29, 2023, from https://blogs.scientificamerican.com/observations/clearing-up-some-misconceptions-about-neurodiversity

Bettin, J. (2019) "The myth of independence: How the social model of disability exposes society's double standards." NeuroClastic, November 11. Accessed on January 29, 2023, from https://neuroclastic.com/celebration-of-interdependence

Dallman, A. R., Williams, K. L., and Villa, L. (2022) "Neurodiversity-affirming practices are a moral imperative for occupational therapy." *The Open Journal of Occupational Therapy 10*, 2, 1–9. https://doi.org/10.15453/2168-6408.1937

Kornblau, B. L. and Robertson, S. M. (2021) "Special issue on occupational therapy with neurodivergent people." *The American Journal of Occupational Therapy 75*, 3. https://doi.org/10.5014/AJOT.2021.753001

Rakshit, D. (2022) "How society's fixation on independence as a universal goal excludes disabled, chronically ill people." *The Swaddle*, August 27. Accessed on January 29, 2023, from https://theswaddle.com/how-societys-fixation-on-independence-as-a-universal-goal-excludes-disabled-chronically-ill-people

Chapter 18, Speech and Language

Cummins, C., Pellicano, E., and Crane, L. (2020) "Autistic adults' views of their communication skills and needs." *International Journal of Language & Communication Disorders 55*, 5, 678–689. https://doi.org/10.1111/1460-6984.12552

DeThorne, L. S. and Gerlach-Houck, H. (2023) "Resisting ableism in school-based speech-language therapy: An invitation to change." *Language, Speech, and Hearing Services in Schools 54*, 1, 1–7. https://doi.org/10.1044/2022_LSHSS-22-00139

DeThorne, L. S., Hengst, J. A., Valentino, H. A., and Russell, S. A. (2015) "More than words: Examining communicative competence through a preschool-age child with autism." *Inclusion 3*, 3, 176–196. https://doi.org/10.1352/2326-6988-3.3.176

Lees, E. (no date) "Neurodivergent-affirming SLT." Autistic SLT. Accessed on January 29, 2023, from www.autisticslt.com/nd-affirmingslt

Richmond, J. and Baicher, V. (2022) "Communicating with neurodivergent patients." Don't Forget The Bubbles. https://doi.org/10.31440/DFTB.48007

Taylor, L. (2022) "Communication styles, counseling, and neurodiversity." *Psychology Today, Australia*, January 11. Accessed on January 29, 2023, from www.psychologytoday.com/au/blog/the-neurodivergent-therapist/202201/communication-styles-counseling-and-neurodiversity

Vance, T. (2021) "Weavers and concluders: Two communication styles no one knows exist." NeuroClastic, April 5. Accessed on January 29, 2023, from https://neuroclastic.com/weavers-and-concluders-two-communication-styles-no-one-knows-exist

Vidal, V., McAllister, A., and DeThorne, L. S. (2020) "Communication profile of a minimally verbal school-age autistic child: A case study." *Language, Speech, and Hearing Services in Schools 51*, 3, 671–686. https://doi.org/10.1044/2020_LSHSS-19-00021

Chapter 19, Play

Burch, J. (2022) "Don't change autistic play. Join in." *ASHA Leader 27*, 6, 22–23. Accessed on February 23, 2023, from https://leader.pubs.asha.org/do/10.1044/leader.MIW.27112022.slp-antiableist-play.22/full

Fanning, P. A. J., Sparaci, L., Dissanayake, C., Hocking, D. R., and Vivanti, G. (2021) "Functional play in young children with autism and Williams syndrome: A cross-syndrome comparison." *Child Neuropsychology 27*, 1, 125–149. https://doi.org/10.1080/09297049.2020.1804846

Gilmore, S., Frederick, L. K., Santillan, L., and Locke, J. (2019) "The games they play: Observations of children with autism spectrum disorder on the school playground." *Autism 23*, 6, 1343–1353. https://doi.org/10.1177/1362361318811987

Hancock, C. L. (2020) "We don't play that way, we play this way: Functional play behaviours of children with autism and severe learning difficulties." *Research in Developmental Disabilities 103*. https://doi.org/10.1016/J.RIDD.2020.103688

Holmes, E. and Willoughby, T. (2005) "Play behaviour of children with autism spectrum disorders." *Journal of Intellectual & Developmental Disability 30*, 3, 156–164. https://doi.org/10.1080/13668250500204034

Jarrold, C. (2003) "A review of research into pretend play in autism." *Autism 7*, 4, 379–390. https://doi.org/10.1177/1362361303007004004

Libby, S., Powell, S., Messer, D., and Jordan, R. (1998) "Spontaneous play in children with autism: A reappraisal." *Journal of Autism and Developmental Disorders 28*, 6, 487–497. https://doi.org/10.1023/A:1026095910558

Schaefer, C. E. (ed.) (2011) *Foundations of Play Therapy*, Second Edition. New York: John Wiley & Sons Inc.

Schaefer, C. E. and Drewes, A. (2013) *The Therapeutic Powers of Play: 20 Core Agents of Change*, 2nd Edition. New York: John Wiley & Sons Inc.

Chapter 20, A Final Reflection

No references.

Index